THE
LOW-BACK
REPAIR MANUAL

5 Lessons for Finally Taking Control of Your Low-Back Pain

CRAIG PEARLBERG

PEARLFIT, LLC
Victor, NY

The Low-Back Repair Manual
5 Lessons for Finally Taking Control of your Low-Back Pain

Original "Pelvic Tilt" sketch by Alison Garrity
Cover design by Ioana Naniş
Editing and interior design by Sara Zibrat
Royalty-free illustrations from www.123rf.com
All photos © Craig Pearlberg

DISCLAIMER: This book is only intended as a reference. The author and publisher of this book and its associated materials have used their best efforts to ensure their accuracy. The spine and its supporting structures are very complicated and there are a number of factors that can lead to long-term pain.

    The Low-Back Repair Manual attempts to specifically deal with the underlying muscular support structure for your lower back. The author and publisher make no representations or warranties with respect to the completeness of the contents of this material and shall in no event be held liable for any adverse effects resulting from the use or application of the information contained herein.

    All back pain should be discussed with you doctor. Always consult your doctor before starting any exercise program.

ISBN: 978-0-9973579-0-5

Library of Congress Control Number: 2016943487

Publisher's Cataloging-in-Publication Data
(Prepared by The Donohue Group, Inc.)

Names: Pearlberg, Craig.
Title: The low-back repair manual : 5 lessons for finally taking control of your low-back pain / Craig Pearlberg.
Other Titles: Low back repair manual
Description: Victor, NY : Pearlfit, LLC, [2016] | Includes bibliographical references.
Identifiers: LCCN 2016943487 | ISBN 978-0-9973579-0-5
Subjects: LCSH: Backache--Exercise therapy. | Back--Movements. | Human locomotion. | Posture.
Classification: LCC RD771.B217 P43 2016 | DDC 617.5/64062--dc23

Published by PEARLFIT, LLC
Victor, NY
USA

This paper meets the requirements of ANSI/NISO 239.48-1992 (Permanence of Paper).

*This book is for anyone who deals
with low-back pain and the problems it
brings to your life.
Moving smarter and living stronger
are finally within reach!*

Acknowledgements

Thanks to Phil D., Kevin, Teri, John, Phil S., Rick,
Cheryl, Joan, Jasna, Don and Justin for all your support.

Thanks to Dad, Jeff and Jerry for
always asking the tough questions.

Thanks to my mom for
mixing optimism with the right dose of reality.

Thanks to my daughter, Emerson,
for helping to keep me young and totally inspired.

And thanks to Susan, for giving me all the love and
support that a wonderful wife can give. I love you, deeply.

Table of Contents

About the Author

After spending most of my life making one unhealthy decision after another, I finally decided it was time to take care of my own poor health. A 20-year smoker, chronic over-eater, and sufferer of persistent low-back "attacks," my change began by simply committing to a short walk each day, and six months later I completed my first marathon!

Running wasn't enough to keep my back pain at bay, so I continued the long journey of learning about—and improving—my own personal health. The next step was to certify as a Personal Trainer through the American Council on Exercise. However, I wanted to understand even more about how to get healthy and stay that way, so I eventually earned ACE's Health Coach certification and I am now specifically trained as a Corrective Exercise Specialist.

As I approach 50 years of age, I am in the best overall health of my life. Regular exercise and good diet have played a big role, but I would not feel nearly as good if I didn't pay attention to moving correctly and caring for my muscles. Years after I started down a healthier road, I began to fully understand the many components that contributed to my back troubles and—after working with many clients, doing constant research and continuing my practice of healthy movement—I developed the strategies in this manual that will enable you to finally take control of your low-back pain, too.

Glossary

General Terms

Back attack: The acute or most painful phase of back pain, which "takes you out" or significantly limits your activity for a period of time.

Spasm, seizure: Although these terms refer to slightly different actions within the muscles, I use them interchangeably in this manual.

Cervical spine: Neck area.

Thoracic spine: Mid back.

Lumbar spine: Lower back.

Pelvis: the entire basin-like, bony structure near the base of the spine; it attaches the legs to the torso.

Hips: In general, the term "hips" refers to the wider sides of the pelvis, from the waist to the thigh. It also sometimes refers to the joint where the thigh bone (femur) and pelvis meet, aka the "hip joint."

Reps: Short for "repetitions." It indicates how many times in a row you need to repeat the *same* activity.

Sets: A set is a group of reps. For example, 2 sets of 10 means one set of ten reps, followed by another set of ten reps (usually with a specific rest period in between).

Pack your shoulders: the practice of tucking your shoulders down and back to ensure that they're kept in the correct position for maximum stability and safety during all movements.

Body, bodies, our bodies, your body: I use these terms interchangeably, but ultimately, I really mean the body that you live in.

Floor, ground, yoga mat: Take your pick, unless otherwise noted.

Fascia: The connective tissue that binds/covers all the internal muscles and organs of the body.

Soft tissue: Basically, whatever is not bone (i.e. muscles, tendons, fascia, and organs).

Muscle Names

The muscles listed below are defined in more detail in Lesson One, but—for the sake of clarity—I'm including a quick summary. At times, generic terms are used for specific muscles, for example, butt muscles = glutes. There are hundreds of muscles in our bodies and this manual is not intended to be a comprehensive lesson in human anatomy.

Abdominals, Abs: These terms usually refer to the **Rectus Abdominis** and **Obliques.** The rectus abdominis is the most common abdominal muscle we think of and is the one that runs up and down the front of the body. The obliques sit beneath the rectus abdominis (deeper under the skin) and work at opposite angles to each other.

Transverse Abdominal, TVA: It is officially one of the muscles in the abdominal group, but I'll also refer to it separately in these lessons. It wraps around your body, beneath the rectus abdominis and obliques.

Back Extensors: A group of back muscles running beside the spine from the pelvis to the neck. Although there are many more muscles in your back, when I use the generic term "back muscles," I'm referring to this group. They are also known as the erector spinae muscles.

Hip Flexors: A group that can contain many different muscles in the front and sides of the hip. However, for this manual, I'm specifically referring to the two that attach from the lumbar spine and pelvis and connect to the top of the femur. This group also includes one of the four quadriceps muscles (see below).

Rectus Femoris: One of the four quadriceps muscles, it is the only one of the "quads" with major involvement at the hips and pelvis; it runs down the front of the thigh.

Gluteus Maximus: The larger butt muscle. Also referred to as **Glute or Glutes**.

Hamstrings: The three muscles on the back of the thigh.

Introduction

Everyone knows somebody with low-back pain. In the U.S. alone, 80% of adults experience back pain at some point in their lives[1] and low-back pain is the leading cause of disability worldwide.[2] In fact, it's very likely that you (or someone you care about) are dealing with nagging, uncontrolled low-back pain and that needs to change. Also, if you're like me and millions of others, you've probably spent a lot of time and money trying to keep that pain (and its effects on your family and your life) to a minimum.

However, if you're reading this book, you've probably decided that just hearing or reading about "basic preventative measures," taking painkillers, and visiting multiple doctors isn't enough. You need something more: concrete and ready-to-use lessons on how to finally take control of your low-back pain. That's what this manual is all about.

The Low-Back Repair Manual will quickly allow you to:

- Better understand and manage the underlying muscular causes of your back issues.

1. American Chiropractic Association. *Back Pain Facts and Statistics.* Retrieved May 2, 2015, from acatoday.org
2. D. Hoy, L. March, P. Brooks, A, Woolf, C. Bain, G. Williams, et al. (2014, March). The Global Burden of Low Back Pain: Estimates from the Global Burden of Disease 2010 Study. *Annals of the Rheumatic Diseases,* 968-974.

- Immediately gain more strength to move through work, life or play.

- Lose the fear that, at any minute, you could be "taken out" by a low-back spasm, seizure, or what I call a "back attack".

Let me first tell you what brought me to this point and how I came to be in a unique position to help you. You see, not only am I a corrective exercise specialist, trained specifically to understand how to get people moving smarter and living stronger when faced with an injury, but I am also a long-time sufferer of low-back attacks.

My first attack hit me over 30 years ago while I was shoveling the driveway, and it laid me up for several days. Being a teenager, my body was still young enough to recover quickly. However, as I explain in this manual, the older we get, the more our bodies become susceptible to breakdown and low-back pain, and the longer it can take to fully recover. My back attacks kept coming and started causing enough trouble to make a significant impact on my life. In fact, I originally became certified as a personal trainer through the American Council on Exercise just to get a grip on my own health. It took many years of research, practice, and working with clients to finally be ready to share this information with you now.

It's important that you go through each lesson in this book in order. If you want to experience this massive change in your life, there are some concepts and theories you need to understand before jumping into movement practices and exercises.

The Low-Back Repair Manual will teach you how your lower back, pelvis and hip area (known as the lumbo-pelvic-hip region) is designed by nature to support and stabilize movement. These lessons explain why this area can cause so much trouble and pain, and will show you how to make use of your body's natural support system to move more safely through life. You'll then know what to do to avoid back attacks and to stay strong, confident and pain-minimized.

I use the term "pain-minimized" for a specific reason. Notice that the subtitle of this book is "5 Lessons for Finally Taking Control of Your Low-Back Pain." It doesn't say "Get Rid of Low-Back Pain Forever" or "Never Be Bothered by Low-Back Pain Again." For a number of reasons, ridding yourself of low-back pain forever is very difficult to do.[3]

Once low-back struggles begin, you can be faced with a lifetime of battles to manage the pain and keep yourself strong and stable. However, if you follow the lessons and instructions I lay out in this book, you will have the blueprint for consistently winning those battles. I cannot promise you a pain-free future, but the steps you take now can keep your future low-back pain—and its life-limiting effects—to a minimum.

After incorporating this knowledge into your life, you can begin to eliminate missed workdays, continue to play with your kids, and generally move through life without the fear of being "laid up" by a painful or disabling back seizure.

---

3. Anthony D. Woolf and Bruce Pfleger (2003). Burden of major musculoskeletal conditions. Bulletin of the World Health Organization, 81, p. 652.

In Lesson One, *Awareness*, you'll learn about what's happening in your body that leads to low-back pain over the long term. I'll go through the muscular and skeletal anatomy of the section of our bodies that we call "the core," as well as what purpose the core really serves.

We'll dig deeper into your core in Lesson Two, *The Transverse Abdominis*, to learn about this important muscle. Understanding how to isolate and activate the TVA is critical for maintaining a strong and stable body and will allow you to take advantage of the rest of the book.

In Lesson Three, *Posture Makes Perfect*, you'll use the knowledge of core anatomy and activation to get yourself into a good, old-fashioned, standing posture, just like they taught you when you were younger. Knowing the differences between good and bad posture is a great beginning; consistently practicing and maintaining good posture is the best and simplest strengthening exercise you can do to minimize low-back pain.

As you get to Lesson Four, *Moving Smarter with Positional Postures*, you'll be on your way to living stronger through work, life or play. You'll learn to use the core to support your back while correctly maneuvering through all of the potentially dangerous activities of life, such as getting up and down from the floor, lifting, getting out of bed, twisting and leaning over. This is where the serious attention and practice begins to enable you to live your life without fear and avoid back trouble over the long term.

That practice continues in Lesson Five, as you learn to start *Achieving Muscle Balance*. This final lesson teaches you the valuable techniques and exercises needed to keep your core and low-back muscles strong, flexible, and in balance for years of active living.

This manual is not a complete and exhaustive explanation of the topic of low-back pain, but I intend to provide more than enough education for anyone to become immediately stronger, more confident, and pain-minimized. If you follow the lessons and do your own core activation, positional posture and exercise practice, you can turn your life around. Instead of your low-back pain controlling you, you can finally take control of your low-back pain.

Lesson 1: Awareness

What's Happening in Our Bodies

Most of the time you might experience your back pain as just a dull reminder to "stretch" the tightness you feel. Too often, that tight muscle turns into nagging pain, an immovable muscle and eventually—at what seems like a random moment—it might spasm or cramp painfully. You may be lucky enough to only have "some" back pain "now and then," or perhaps you've already had one or two disabling "back attacks." Either way, there's a good chance you've been wearing down your body in ways you wouldn't be aware of until it's too late.

Micro Traumas

In their *Book of Body Maintenance and Repair*, the American Physical Therapy Association states:

> "...If there is no obvious cause for pain, the culprit is often the accumulated stress, strain and abuse from years of poor posture and body mechanics."[4]

This slow, day-by-day breaking down of our bodies from normal use and gravity can create what are called

---

4. Marilyn Moffat and Steve Vickery (1999). *American Physical Therapy Association Book of Body Maintenance and Repair.* New York, NY: Henry Holt.

micro traumas. That stress is compounded by the short-term and long-term trouble we experience from a lack of strength and the imbalances in our muscles that stem from "side-dominance" and improper mechanics.

Every minute of every day, our bodies are slowly breaking down because of the regular activity of living, and it's inevitable that slight irritations of the muscle or fascia tissue occur over time. In fact, improving strength depends on the minor breakdown and repair of tissues, and short-term inflammation plays an important role in this process.

However, if not managed correctly, this can lead to scarring and long-term inflammation, which results in a reduction of the tissues' range of motion. In time, this decreases flexibility, strength and function. All of this creates an environment of "danger" for joints, muscles and other soft tissue, which could lead to a muscle going into emergency protection mode by spasming or cramping painfully, and BAM! You're out of commission.

Even if you've had an impact injury at some point, but were "cleared" by your doctor with no evident skeletal damage, or if you are currently dealing with disc issues, arthritis, stenosis or one of the many other skeletal issues, your muscles can tighten up to protect your spine (and themselves) and continue to cause nagging pain.

Also, if you've had spinal surgery for one of these skeletal problems, it's possible that soft tissues and bones adjacent to the repair are taking on more work than they were designed for[5] and the resulting overuse can lead to a nagging long-term problem.

To be clear, each person's back pain is unique. There can be multiple and various factors that influence back pain and the problems increase from age thirty into the mid-sixties.[6] One major contributing factor is continually using poor body mechanics. After all, a bulging disc does not usually occur out of nowhere and stenosis or arthritis doesn't develop in a single day.

The differences from person to person make it hard to offer a single remedy that works for everyone, but I discovered that if you learn about and focus consistent awareness on some key muscles, and consistently move your body correctly, your lower back can keep you strong and upright for years of active living.

A Lack of Strength

Physical strength is what makes all of the movements of daily life possible. Flexibility and balance are important, but without strength to hold us up and allow us to bear the

5.   Kristen E. Radcliff, MD, Christopher K. Kepler, MD, Andre Jakoi, MD, Gursukhman S. Sidhu, MBBS, Jeffery Rihn, MD, Alexander R. Vaccaro, MD, PhD, Todd J. Albert, MD, Alan S. Hilibrand, MD (2013). Adjacent segment disease in the lumbar spine following different treatment interventions. *The Spine Journal, 13* (10), 1339–1349.
6.   D. Hoy, P. Brooks, F. Blyth and R. Buchbinder. (2010, December). The epidemiology of low back pain. *Best Practice & Research Clinical Rheumatology*, 769-781.

load of whatever we're doing, we'd all be useless heaps on the floor ...or couch.

There are different ways of measuring strength. We can talk about the burst of power needed to push your car out of the snow or to pick up a child to hold; the muscle endurance needed to hold that child or carry groceries; and the pure strength you need to handle a heavy load. As you can imagine, lacking any of these types of strength can impact your life in a variety of ways.

For the purpose of these lessons, we're talking about endurance: the endurance to hold ourselves upright, stay in motion, and maintain long-term strength to last throughout the day and throughout our lives. We're also concerned with the effects that weak muscles (such as the commonly weak abdominals or gluteals) have on our pelvic stability. As you read on, you'll also begin to see how this lack of strength can be so debilitating and lead to chronic back pain.

Muscle Imbalance

There are different muscle imbalances that can affect low-back pain. The one that we're most familiar with is right-side or left-side dominance. We've all experienced this "sided" imbalance in one form or another, as your "dominant" side muscles are stronger and often tighter. These are sometimes referred to as "hypertonic" muscles. This means that they have too much tension or strength and can lead to (or even be caused by) weaker and looser muscles ("hypotonic") on the non-dominant side.

Another imbalance—and one that is strongly stressed in this manual—is when muscles that are meant to work with (or against) each other are out of balance. These muscular relationships are vital to our overall strength and stability. This point will become much clearer in the Anatomy section, as we explore how the pull of a strong, tight muscle group can create a serious problem when counteracted by a weak, loose one.

Anatomy

Spine Structure

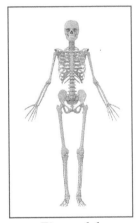

Figure 1-1

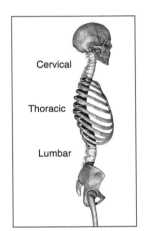

Figure 1-2

The image of a skeleton, like the one in Figure 1-1, is probably something everyone has seen at some point in their lives, but I want to highlight some important facts. I want you to take note of the three main curves in the spine, as illustrated in Figure 1-2. You're probably all familiar with these curves, but it's important to keep in mind that they each evolved for the same critical reason: to help us balance our weight.

The curve is the body's ingenious way of distributing the pressure we experience from gravity, various postures, and all of our daily movements (think of the great strength of the arch in nature and architecture). We're born with a thoracic curve, but the other two don't develop until they're needed. The cervical curve develops as we practice and then succeed in holding up our heads (which is one reason "tummy time" is so important for babies). The lumbar curve forms as we build the strength and skills needed to stand on our own two feet.

This single point about the lumbar curve highlights the great importance of this part of the body, because it reinforces the fact that we need a strong lumbar spine in order to be stable in an upright position. It distributes the weight and pressure of so much of the activity in our daily lives. However, if you look at the skeleton in Figure 1-1, you can see there are no bones or other structures supporting this most vital area. The cervical spine is also without other supporting bones, but it only handles the weight of your head.

The lower back is part of the vital connection between our legs and torso and should be our center of gravity and all movement. It is completely dependent on the soft tissues that exist in this area for support. In fact, this area of the body is so important that we call it (with all of its muscles, bones and attachments) the "core."

What, Exactly, Is the Core?

The core is not just the abs we've all come to know and love ... or hate. And it's not just a mysterious group of muscles so often referred to by health and fitness enthusiasts. It is also so much more than a "six pack."

Many people have heard the word "core," and have a general idea of the function and location of the core of our bodies, but they usually don't understand what its physical structure is or, most importantly, how to activate and use it to remain strong and on your feet day after day. This idea of how to find and use the core (which we'll explore in detail) is a critical point for both this manual and for your life.

Essentially, the core is the midsection of the body, and its purpose is to support and stabilize our bodies during movement and exertion. It is vital for transferring energy from the lower body to the upper body (for example, when pushing furniture into place or swinging a golf club).

In general, the core consists of groups of muscles that extend from the diaphragm down to the upper legs, although at any given point many different muscles may be contracting to stabilize the body during a given movement. Some deep back muscles get involved, along with the all-important muscles that attach to the hips and pelvis.

These all-important muscles include the hamstrings and gluteals (Figure 1-3), hip flexors (Figure 1-4), back

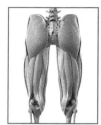 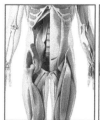 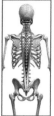 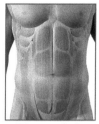 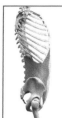

Figure 1-3   Figure 1-4   Figure 1-5   Figure 1-6   Figure 1-7

extensors (Figure 1-5), the well-known abs (Figure 1-6), and the mother of all core muscles (the one that we'll stress the most in these lessons), the Transverse Abdominis (TVA, Figure 1-7).

There are entire courses dedicated to our muscle anatomy but, for our needs, I'm touching briefly on some of the functions of individual muscles and muscle groups, how they are sparked into action, as well as what bones they attach to. These points are important because, when we misuse or overuse our bodies, the muscles and bones can be pulled out of alignment.[7]

Although very small, this pull on a muscle can create a corresponding tug on another attached or adjacent muscle. As with the issue of side-dominance I mentioned earlier, this muscular balancing act, coupled with the development of micro traumas and the way muscle nerves respond to strain, creates an environment for potential pain.

---

7.   American Council on Exercise (2010). *ACE's Essentials of Exercise Science for Fitness Professionals.* (C. X. Brayant and D. J. Green, eds.) San Diego, CA: American Council on Exercise.

Within the Muscle at Work

Since the whole point of these lessons is to learn how to finally control your low-back pain, and managing your muscles is a big part of that, it's important to explain a few points about how our muscles work. There are three kinds of muscles in the body—skeletal, smooth and cardiac—and this manual deals only

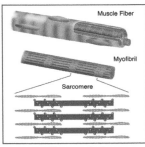

Figure 1-8

with skeletal muscles. These are the muscles that attach to the skeleton, but they are also known as voluntary muscles because we have voluntary control of them.

Merriam-Webster.com defines a "spasm" as "a sudden, uncontrolled and often painful tightening of a muscle ... a sudden and usually brief occurrence of something you cannot control." They are mostly activated by an irritation to a nerve that sends an emergency signal to the muscle.

Each muscle contains thousands of muscle fiber bundles held in place by layers of fascia. Within those fibers are groups of two different protein filaments (Sarcomeres, Figure 1-8). These filaments line up next to each other and run along the length of the muscle in line with whichever direction that muscle moves or contracts. Through a chemical reaction, the nerves signal those protein filaments to pull on each other, resulting in a contraction and creating the force we know of as muscle strength.

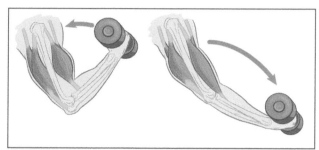

Figure 1-9: Bicep Curl, showing concentric and eccentric contraction

It's important to remember that, not only can a muscle be contracting to create force while shortening (concentric muscle contraction), but it can also contract while lengthening (eccentric contraction). Figure 1-9 shows this idea using the bicep curling action. As you curl the weight towards your shoulder, the bicep muscle (on the front of the upper arm) shortens while creating the force needed to lift the weight. The muscle still has to work against gravity as the weight is lowered back down and, in order to do this, it must continue to produce force while lengthening.

This comes into play in our lives when we bend forward at the waist and the muscles in the back of our legs and buttocks are lengthening at the same time they are working hard to keep us from falling over. But if that particular muscle group isn't strong enough (and it often isn't), other muscles around the pelvis and lower back have to do much more work than they're built for. And that, as you can imagine, can lead to trouble.

It can go even deeper, as is the case when a muscle senses danger to the bone or joint it connects to. For example, in the case of some back pain, the smallest spinal muscles may sense a disc being dangerously squeezed or shifting out of place and will seize tightly in an effort to "splint" the danger.[8]

A seizure in one of these small muscles can have a ripple effect on larger, adjacent ones, which can cause a more widespread muscular response. Unfortunately, the problem can persist when the muscles fail to relax and continue to "splint" long after the "danger" passes.[9]

We need to be careful when trying to force a muscle to relax, or push through a stretch, as there are over-excited nerves at work and they're on high alert for more danger. Two reflex mechanisms, or receptors, are on duty to tell the nerve to either freak out or chill out. Put simply, one of those receptors works against a stretch and the other allows it to continue. If one of these receptors sense danger from a rapid or unacceptable muscle contraction, it fires that protection signal and BAM! You're seized up.

The Under-Appreciated SI Joint

The point at the base of the spine (where the upper body attaches to the lower) is called the sacroiliac joint, or SI joint. The sacrum is the lowest part of the spine and the ilium is the wide bone that is part of the pelvis. The SI joint is where they come together, and is named for the parts it joins: "sacro-" and "iliac" refer to the sacrum and ilium.

---

8.   Phil Dodge, DC. (2015, July 1). Facet joint anatomy and function. [Personal interview].
9.   Ibid.

As you start to learn how the important muscle groups connect to and support the lumbo-pelvic hip complex, it becomes easy to understand how the SI joint is so susceptible to strain.

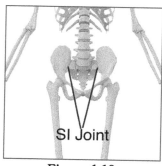

Figure 1-10

I believe that this spot (where the pelvis is connected to the lumbar and sacral spine) is at the heart of so many of our low-back issues. The SI joint, along with the lower back, has to support most of the weight of our upper body, which can be 65% or more of our overall body weight. It has to allow (or give support to) a huge variety of movements—some of which it's designed for and some not so much. It is a strong joint with little movement, but it still has to act as a tremendous pivot point, not just between the upper and lower parts of our body, but also between the four major muscle groups that attach to the hips, pelvis and spine.

The Body's Connections

There are various types of tissue that connect the different parts of our bodies and it will be helpful to identify a few of them. The *ligaments* connect bone to bone and are flexible enough to allow joints to move around but strong enough to also help hold those joints together. The Anterior Cruciate Ligament (ACL) and Medial Collateral Ligament (MCL) of the knee are commonly known examples of ligaments.

Tendons attach muscle to bone. They are extremely strong and inflexible and help to signal impending injury to muscle nerves, which, in turn, signal muscle fibers to contract for protection. The Achilles tendon, which attaches the two calf muscles to the heel, is an important and well-known example of a tendon.

As far as these lessons are concerned, the most important connective tissue is what's called *fascia*. Much is still being learned about fascia and it could be discussed in much greater detail. However, for our purposes, I'm just saying what is necessary to show how this important connective tissue plays a big role in maintaining healthy movement and minimizing pain.

The fascia in our bodies is essentially a very large, single piece of tissue. It not only wraps and protects all interior structures (bones, organs, muscles and nerves) like a sheath, but also helps control movement and conveys information about our balance, position and overall internal health.[10] There are multiple layers of this tissue throughout the body, and major connections at certain points (the lumbar and abdominal areas, for example) to give added strength, stability and flexibility. If the fascia becomes tight or "bound up," it can restrict our muscles and movements.[11]

As you can see, the muscles and connective tissues in your body act as the support and security protecting the

10 Justin Price (2009). *Understanding Muscles and Movement*. Space Café Media.
11 American Council on Exercise (2010), op. cit.

skeleton and holding it in place. This demanding, life-long effort of the muscles, together with potential imbalances and weakness from the everyday stress of moving through life, have led to some degree of back pain in nearly 80% of adults.[12]

While you might now begin to understand how the structures in our core help keep us strong and upright, as you progress through this manual, you'll see even more clearly that learning how to manage this soft tissue support network can give you the skills for finally taking control of your low-back pain.

---

12   National Institute of Neurological Disorders and Stroke. (2014, December). *Low Back Pain Fact Sheet*. Retrieved December 2014, from National Institute of Neurological Disorders and Stroke: http://www.ninds.nih.gov/disorders/backpain/   detail_backpain. htm#3102_4

The Pelvic Tilt

As I mentioned in the previous section, many of the core muscles attach to the pelvis and hips. Because of this, the stability of the pelvis itself is critical for low-back health. In the following sections, you'll learn more about these important muscles but, for now, take a close look at Figure 1-11.

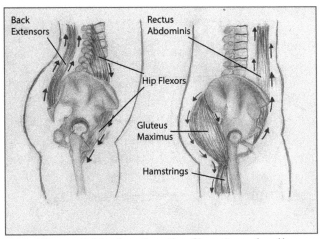

Figure 1-11, showing the direction of pull
for the muscles that affect pelvic tilt

So much of what's contained in these pages comes down to managing the tilt of your pelvis, which is achieved through the balance and control of the four key muscle groups highlighted in Figure 1-11 (for our purposes, the gluteus maximus and hamstrings are considered a single group). The arrows show in which direction the muscle pulls when contracted.

You'll usually see three terms used when referring to a pelvic tilt. To help illustrate them, I want you to think of your pelvis as a basin of water. If you tip the basin *forward* to pour water over your toes, then you're putting the pelvis into an "anterior" (or forward) tilt. If you wanted to pour the water down the back of your legs, you'd create a "posterior," or backward, tilt. And if you wanted the water to stay *in* the basin, you would keep your pelvis in a *neutral* position, not tipped in either direction.

As you can see on the left of Figure 1-11, the pelvis is in a slight anterior tilt. The directional arrows show that this is caused by the back extensors pulling up from behind while the hip flexors tug down along the front. The resulting tilt causes the hip joint to flex (pushes the hip joint back) and increases the lumbar curve. The image on the right shows the rectus abdominis, glutes and hamstrings drawing the pelvis into a slight posterior tilt. This extends the hip (forces the hip joint forward) and flattens the low-back (lumbar) curve.

Because an excessive tilt can have significant, adverse effects on the lumbar spine, a fundamental practice for most people with low-back pain is to keep the pelvis in a neutral position, as this puts the lumbar spine into its proper curve. For many, that means reversing an anterior tilt that's caused by tight hip flexors and strong back muscles pulling on the pelvis, but not being effectively counteracted by weak abs, glutes and hamstrings. In fact, just actively squeezing your butt muscles can go a long way to pulling the pelvis back into neutral and stabilizing your lower back.

Let's get into more detail about those muscle groups and, as you read through the next pages, refer back to the pelvic tilt image, if needed.

Abdominals

Figure 1-12 shows the muscle most people think of when they hear the word "abs": the rectus abdominis. It is the long muscle in the front of the belly and has a main purpose of bringing the chest towards the hips, which is what happens when you bend your spine forward. However, it *also* functions to slow down the spine from arching too far backwards,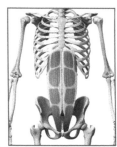

Figure 1-12

which is what can happen when serving a tennis ball or reaching up to put dishes away.

To accomplish its work, it has attachments at the bottom of the pelvis (the pubic bone) all the way up to where the ribs come together in the area called the sternum. It also connects to a few of the lower front ribs. The location of these attachments creates an upward pull from the bottom front of the pelvis, which has the effect of tilting the pelvis backwards.

The *obliques* also have an impact on stability. There are internal and external obliques on each side of the torso. Both work to assist in bending sideways and also toward the front of our body, while simultaneously resisting the opposite side's movements, in order to keep us from falling over. They also help to compress the abdomen for support and stronger breathing and are vital for rotating the torso.

The *internal* obliques (Figure 1-13) stretch from the front of the bottom three ribs and the top of the pelvis and extend around to the back of the torso near the spine. Their muscle fibers are lined up as though they are stretching into your back pockets. The external obliques (Figure 1-14) work from the opposite angle; they attach from the sides of the lower eight ribs to the front of the abdomen. They line up as though reaching into your front pockets.

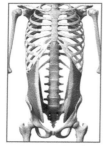   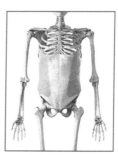

Figure 1-13   Figure 1-14
Internal Obliques   *External Obliques*

Back Extensors (Erector Spinae Group)

There are several different muscles in this group, with different attachments and slightly different purposes. To keep this lesson as simple as possible (and because they all play similar stabilizing roles), I'm going to discuss them as though they were one muscle.

Generally speaking, they attach to the top of the pelvis and the fascia in our lower and middle back, and then travel along the back of the ribs and spine all the way up to the base of the head. Part of the group also attaches to the lower ribs. The multifidus (Figure 1-18) sits deeper in the body than the other three.

Erector Spinae Group

Figure 1-15	Figure 1-16	Figure 1-17	Figure 1-18
spinalis thoracis	*iliocostalis*	*longissimus*	*multifidus*

The main function of this group of muscles is to keep the torso upright and arch it backwards when needed. But it also has the job of lengthening when it's needed to keep us from falling forward, such as when we lean forward over the sink while doing dishes. Because of its deep connections to individual vertebrae, the multifidus also has a primary function of stabilizing and supporting some of the smallest movements of the spine. Because of these different functions, the back extensors are one of those muscle groups that can end up working overtime when its opposing groups aren't strong enough.

For example, when the hamstrings and glutes aren't able to do their "lengthening" work of keeping the upper body above the hips, the back extensors take on extra duty, and that—as you can guess from the theme here—can lead to a nasty pain in the back. And, since this muscle group is connected directly to so much of the spine, it can be negatively affected if the spine is compromised. This adds an even deeper layer of danger.

Gluteus Maximus and Hamstring Group

This group, which works to counteract the back extensors in a pelvic tilt, also has the purpose of "extending the hips." That is, they bring the hips back in line from a forward bent position, creating a posterior pelvic tilt. This is how they attempt to keep the upper body aligned over the hips.

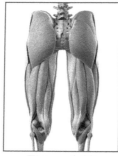

The gluteus maximus is the muscle that gives our butt the definition we've come to know and love. It runs from the back of the pelvis and base of the spine, and then extends along the back of the hip and into the upper part of the thigh bone (femur).

Figure 1-19
Gluteus Maximus & Hamstring Group

The gluteus maximus (or "glute") is one of the largest and strongest muscles in the body but, unfortunately, most of the time it is either weak or chronically inactive. In other words, we spend too much time sitting on our butt and not enough time putting our butt muscles to work! Eventually, they fail to activate when needed and our backs pay the price.

Working in sync with the glutes to pull the pelvis in place, the hamstrings play a major role in the stability of the pelvis and the pain in our backs. They primarily attach to the "sitting bones" (ischial tuberosity), run along the back of the thigh bone, cross the knee and connect to either the inside or outside of the top of the lower leg. Due to all the sitting we do, and/or the fact that we unconsciously lock our knees while standing, the hamstrings are typically weak and/or tight, causing either an unwanted pull on the back and abs, or an insufficient counter-pull against a tight back and the hip flexor group.

Hip Flexors

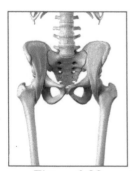 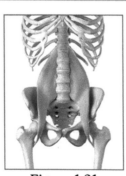 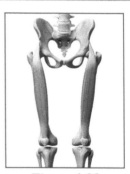

Figure 1-20	Figure 1-21	Figure 1-22
iliacus	*psoas major*	*rectus femoris*

The final group in our pelvic puzzle is made up of several different muscles, but for our purposes we're focused on two that join together at the back of the femur. One of them (the iliacus, shown in Figure 1-20) originates on the inside of the front of the pelvis (*inside* the "basin") while the other (the psoas major—the "p" is silent when pronounced) originates above the pelvis, on the lumbar spine (Figure 1-21). These connections allow for the important work of flexing the hip. Flexing the hip pulls the lumbar spine and pelvis forward into an anterior tilt, while causing the hip joint to shift backward, as though you were taking a bow.

Another key muscle in this group is the rectus femoris (Figure 1-22). This is the largest of the four quadriceps muscles on the front of the thigh. Unlike the other three quad muscles, it has a significant attachment on the pelvis. This attachment makes it an important member of the hip flexor group and its strength and flexibility are vital to the success of controlling your low-back pain.

When trying to do a full sit-up or just getting up from bed, this muscle group tugs the lower back and arches the spine, while it helps to bring the torso towards the legs. The same pull is created when you try to lift your legs while lying on your back. During all of these actions, a strong abdominal group is needed to stabilize the lower back and pelvis against the pull of the flexors. This is just one reason why full sit-ups are dangerous for anyone with low back issues and/or generally weak abs.

While we are sitting, the hip flexors are shortened and this single issue can lead to a lot of low-back pain. If we stay in a seated position for many hours a day, day after day (as so many of us do), those shortened muscles continue to atrophy[13]. In other words, they get even shorter, tighter and/ or weaker over time, and actually lose some of the muscle fibers that simply aren't needed anymore. Eventually, when we try to stand, that tightness creates an unacceptable pull on the lumbar spine, wreaking all kinds of havoc on the pelvis and low-back. Do you see the pattern here?

The Sciatic Problem

Sciatic-related pain is a confusing, tough-to-treat issue, often grouped within the already complex condition of low-back pain. I've included it, not just because some of the pain can be effectively managed by following these lessons, but also because it's common enough to warrant some clarification and suggestions.

The term "sciatica" refers to the symptoms—pain, tingling and numbness—associated with a problem stemming from the sciatic nerve. More specifically, "sciatica" is itself a symptom of one of many possible underlying conditions: bulging or degenerating discs, stenosis, spondylolisthesis, SI joint dysfunction or piriformis syndrome, for example. These are some of the same skeletal problems that can lead to muscle imbalances and spasms of the lower back. To complicate matters more, multiple causes can be occurring simultaneously.

---

13. Sue E. Huether and Kathryn L. McCance, (2004). *Understanding Pathophysiology* (3rd edition). St. Louis, MO: Mosby.

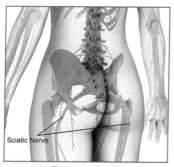

Figure 1-23
Sciatic Nerves

The sciatic nerves emerge from the lower lumbar spine as two small bundles of nerve "roots" (Figure 1-23). These roots travel down along the back of the pelvis, where they join together to form the sciatic nerves, which are the longest and thickest nerves in the body. Then they pass downward through the buttocks and extend down the back of the leg, where they split again and continue downward to the feet. The path these nerves follow through the body, combined with the possible skeletal issues, tend to make this a difficult problem for health care providers and patients to resolve.

For example, on its way through the buttock, the sciatic nerve typically passes directly behind the piriformis muscle, which is a small muscle deep beneath the glute that stretches from the pelvis to the femur. In some people, the nerve actually passes straight through this muscle or even in front of it. Either way, if the piriformis spasms or seizes up, it can significantly irritate the nerve. Careful massaging, stretching and strengthening of the muscles can have a good effect in such cases.

An instance where these techniques may not relieve the pain of sciatica is when spinal stenosis is the cause. The narrowing of the spaces in the spine (which is the hallmark of stenosis) can cause a direct impingement on the nerves. The nerve roots that travel through the lumbar spine are particularly susceptible to this issue. Again, strengthening and balancing the muscles surrounding the troubled section of the spine is still valuable but, in the end, the stenosis must be dealt with if it continues to damage the nerve. (By the way, stenosis can also cause a separate but painful back spasm, which can be very effectively managed with the techniques in this manual).

With the kind of low-back pain I discuss throughout this manual, the muscle spasms are a result of a nerve sending a signal to the muscle. Whatever skeletal issue might be involved, the spasm or "back attack" happens at one or more of the muscles, which is why these lessons are so helpful. With sciatic-related pain, however, the nerve itself is irritated; it may not necessarily affect a muscle. However, although it may not nag at you for years like low-back pain does, direct impingement of a nerve is hard to live with.

Sciatica can take anywhere from a few days to a few months or more to go away but, in any case, I strongly recommend strengthening and balancing the area around the underlying skeletal problem. It's also beneficial to be treated by a good chiropractor and massage therapist. Whether there's a skeletal or muscular condition underlying your sciatic-related pain, there's a great likelihood that making use of these specialists, along with doing your own work as described in this manual, can minimize the discomfort and keep you on the move.

A Little More about Pain

I've made it clear that this manual is about achieving better control over the muscular issues contributing to, and associated with, your low-back pain, but these lessons would not be complete without going a little further into the nature of pain, itself.

The International Association for the Study of Pain (IASP) established a simple definition, which states that pain is:

> "An unpleasant sensory and emotional experience associated with actual or potential tissue damage, or described in terms of such damage."[14]

This definition may be a concise one that we can all agree upon, but it covers a lot of ground. For example, the difference between acute and chronic pain, is an important point to highlight.

Acute pain can be sharp or dull, severe or mild, and usually starts with an incident of some sort (a burn, flu shot, or post-operative condition). It might last for a few minutes or a few months, but it goes away within six months or once the initial cause has stopped occurring or healed. Pain is generally considered to be chronic when it continues for more than six months. or if it persists even

---

14. IASP Taxonomy. International Association for the Study of Pain, 22 May 2012. Web. 24 May 2015. http://www.iasp-pain.org/Taxonomy#Pain

though the underlying cause no longer exists.

As I've mentioned, our nerves are in control of the actions of our muscles. They are also responsible for conveying the unpleasant sensations of pain from within those muscles, as well as from any other place within the body. Whether it's a stomachache, toothache or backache, none of it would be experienced as pain without the signaling that goes on throughout the pathways of our nerves. Broadly speaking, these pathways make up the peripheral and central nervous systems. The central nervous system is contained in the brain and spine, and the peripheral system runs through the rest of the body.

Whenever there is a painful stimulation of a peripheral nerve, as occurs with a cut, burn, toothache or backache, the signal is sent to the spine and up to the brain, where it's processed in a variety of ways. An article by William W. Deardorff, PhD published on www.spine-health.com[15], gives a great example of the variations in pain processing.

In his explanation of Melzack and Wall's Gate Control theory of pain,[16] Deardorff describes a clothespin being clipped onto someone's skin. At first the pain is acute and intense. But, as time passes, the discomfort from the very same stimulus decreases significantly as the brain begins

---

15. William W. Deardorff, PhD, ABPP (2003, March 11). *The Gate Control Theory of Modern Pain*. Retrieved from spine-health. com:http://www.spine-health.com/conditions/chronic-pain/ gate-control-theory-chronic-pain-action
16. R. Melzack, and P. D. Wall (1965). Pain Mechanisms: A New _ Theory. *Science, 150* (3699), 971-979.

to perceive the pain as non-harmful:

> "The brain knows that the clothespin is not causing any injury. Therefore, the brain gradually 'turns the volume down' on the pain message to the point of it being barely noticeable after about thirty minutes. The compression on skin and muscle is still occurring, but it is now perceived as a mild discomfort, if it is noticed at all."[17]

So it's clear that the brain unconsciously manages pain according to the stimulus's importance. But we can also have conscious control over the pain. Notice the use of the word "emotional" in the IASP definition. I think it goes without saying that the low-back pain we experience is so much more than just physical. The nagging, threatening nature of low-back pain, along with its immediate sensations and life-limiting impacts, also makes it very emotional. And—although this emotional response to low-back pain is unique to each individual— a 2005 study showed that:

> "...expectations of decreased pain powerfully reduced both the subjective experience of pain and activation of pain-related brain regions."[18]

17. Deardorff, op. cit.
18. Tetsuo Koyama, John G. McHaffie, Paul J. Laurienti, and Robert C. Coghill (2005). The subjective experience of pain: Where expectations become reality. (E. E. Smith, Ed.) Proceedings of the National Academy of Sciences of the United States of America, 102 (36), 12950–12955.

In other words, simply believing or expecting your pain to be minimized can work to actually minimize your pain. I'm not saying that you can quickly flip a switch in your brain to diminish the pain in your back, but—with the lessons in this manual—not only will you be able to better manage the physical causes, you will also be able to change your emotional response. If you have a positive attitude and expect to have control over your low-back pain, then you'll already be on your way to achieving it.

Lesson 2: The Transverse Abdominis

How It Works

Of all the muscles we've been talking about, it is my belief that the TVA is the most important one in this discussion. Of course it doesn't work on its own, but understanding where it is, what it does, and how and when to put it to work is the single greatest tool you can have in the struggle with nagging low-back pain.

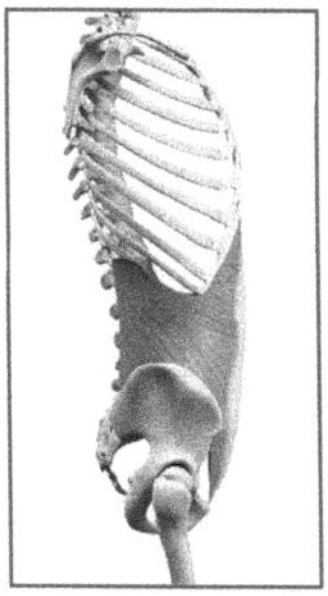

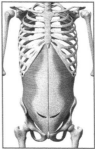

Figure 2-1

Sometimes referred to as our "natural weight-lifting belt," the TVA wraps around our bodies to act like the kind of back brace someone would wear to minimize injury. Its attachments extend all the way around the lower torso—from the lumbar fascia, along the top of the pelvis and over the last six ribs (Figure 2-1), and then around to the front abdominal fascia (Figure 2-2). When activated, the TVA shrinks the diameter of the abdomen by "tightening" the "back brace," in effect compressing the abdomen (this is part of the "sucking in your gut" motion).

Figure 2-2

This compression helps to expel the air from our lungs, push various contents through our organs and—of course—support and stabilize the lumbar spine by creating what's called intra-abdominal pressure. I want to be very

51

clear that to "suck in your gut" and create a useful amount of support for normal activities takes only about 5-10% of the full strength of the TVA.

Some of the practice in these lessons is specifically designed to get that support working on a full-time basis. In other words, the TVA is a muscle that should be gently at work at all times. There are moments when we use much more of its strength, like "bearing down" to give birth or when letting out a strong cough, but this larger amount of pressure can cause injury when it's maintained for long periods of time.

Benefits of an Active TVA

Because the Transverse Abdominis is so critical for low-back stability, keeping it active offers some important benefits. Its conditioning plays a significant role in supporting one of the most important aspects of lower back and full body health—the simple act of good posture. Lightly contracting the muscle helps to give your back the strength to remain in a proper, upright position.

Speaking of strength, the TVA is also a secret weapon of whole body strength and, when it's activated, it can immediately increase the amount of load or weight you can handle. In fact, as you'll see in lesson 4, all movements should start with core activation. To pick up a child, activate the core first; to twist around to the back seat of the car, activate the core first; to just open a door... I think you get the point.

To underscore the importance of starting all movement from the core and—in particular—the TVA, studies have shown that milliseconds before a limb movement, the TVA is automatically activated by a nerve impulse called "feedforward muscle activation." While examining this connection, researchers from the University of Western Australia and Curtin University in Perth, Australia commented:

> "A critical feature of this research is that, in contrast to healthy control subjects, individuals with LBP (low-back pain) do not demonstrate feedforward activity of the TrA (TVA) during rapid limb movements."[19]

There is much more to consider regarding the link between low-back pain and an inefficient or unhealthy nervous system. However, for now it's important to know that simply being aware of the TVA (and knowing how to locate and activate it consistently) is one of the most important keys to preventing and recovering from a back attack and controlling low-back pain in the long term.

How to Activate the TVA

Since the TVA also supports the diaphragm during exhalation, a light cough is often all that's needed to isolate this important stabilizing muscle. Just put your hand on your lower stomach—just below the belly button—and

19. G. Allison, S. Morris, and B. Lay. (2008). *Journal of Orthopaedic and Sports Physical Therapy, 38* (5), 228-237.

cough gently. Close your eyes if you have to, and really try to feel the muscle activate deep within your belly.

For some of you the TVA is activating beneath a thicker belly than you might like, but it *is* happening. There is a muscle in there pushing on the diaphragm to get a good cough going. Now exaggerate the exhale. Let it last for an extra long time and really emphasize it. The longer you hold this action, the more you will feel the muscle working,

Also, if you've ever tried to blow up a balloon, chances are you've pushed from the TVA. You may feel like you're just using your lungs to fill the balloon with air, but they have no muscle and can't work on their own. The rectus abdominis gets involved, but deep in there the transverse abdominis is at work, forcing the air out of your lungs.

Keep It Working

In order to keep your posture correct, your movements safer, and your body stronger, the transverse abdominis must be engaged. Keep it in mind and activate it all of the time—during every step, breath and movement. In fact, to start with right now, try to consciously tilt your pelvis back and forth by lightly contracting the TVA and Rectus Ab. It will help considerably if you also activate your glutes. As you've already learned, the glutes and hamstrings help the abs and TVA tilt the pelvis backwards. If you need to, refer back to the Pelvic Tilt image (Figure 1-11), to help reinforce your understanding of how these muscles act on the pelvis.

Get these muscles working. Alternately contract and relax these muscles and practice putting your pelvis into a neutral position until you recognize it and it becomes very natural. This may take some time, as everyone is unique when it comes to achieving conscious control of some of these muscles, but don't stop working on it, because keeping it working will be a wonderful back saver.

Lesson 3: Posture Makes Perfect

Why Good Posture Is So Good

I think it's a term that we've all heard more than once, and in the next two lessons we're going to put a little "twist" on it. First, though, let's just talk about the benefits of good posture, as well as some bad postures to avoid.

"Good posture" is good for several reasons. You look healthier and stronger, feel more confident[20] and have increased blood flow when sitting or standing up straight.[21] Good posture can allow for deeper breaths by giving more space for the lungs to expand. And—most important for these lessons—maintaining good posture requires gentle, consistent and enduring activation of the key core muscles that keep us so strong and stable and protect against low-back pain. When we keep these muscles working by maintaining good posture, we are, in effect, making them stronger.

Your body is designed to hold a good posture throughout your life and with limited negative side effects. Although you'll definitely feel muscle fatigue when you begin to

---

20. Pablo Briñol, Richard E. Petty, and Benjamin Wagner (2009). Body posture effects on self-evaluation: A self-validation approach. *European Journal of Social Psychology*, 39 (6), 1053-1064.
21. Chiro Economics. (2010, February). *Top 5 consequences to bad posture.* Retrieved from Chiroeco.com

practice a healthy posture, it will eventually feel effortless. This is not only because your muscles will become better conditioned, but also because when the body is correctly aligned above the ground, you're in a position of balance with gravity and the muscles are working minimally.

On the other hand, the cumulative effect of spending too much time in an incorrect posture can be devastating from a musculoskeletal and myofascial perspective. Below, I touch on a few of the most common problems.

Bad Postures, Bad Habits

A Pain in the Neck

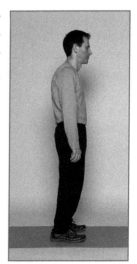

Too much long-term slouching over a computer, smart phone, or other device can cause your head to slowly move forward, leading to what's called "forward head posture." As you can see in Figure 3-1, this is where your head no longer sits over the shoulders supported by the natural cervical curve.

Not only has this been shown to result in a 30% loss in lung capacity,[22] but having a chronically forward head creates a significant strain on your upper back and neck muscles. In fact, for every inch that your head

Figure 3-1

moves forward, it gains 10 pounds of weight, as far as

22. Rene Cailliet and Leonard Gross. (1987). *Rejuvenation Strategy.* New York, NY: Doubleday.

your muscles and tendons are concerned.[23]As Figure 3-1 shows, in order to compensate for the added "weight," the thoracic curve exaggerates in the opposite direction to create balance. Unfortunately, it also puts your skeleton and soft tissue painfully out of balance.

Healthcare providers are also seeing increased cervical issues that some believe are caused by bending one's neck down to read cell phones and tablets. Many of us are familiar with the nagging neck or shoulder pain that can be the warning signs of this ailment, appropriately called "tech neck."

Too Much of a Lower Back Curve

Another common postural deviation is known as excessive lumbar lordosis. This simply means that the lumbar curve has too much... well, curve. This often stems from a pelvis that is tilted too far forward, which can be a critical factor involved in low-back pain.

As I've mentioned, much of the advice out there for minimizing your low-back pain calls for fixing this tilt. Unfortunately, much of that "advice" fails to explain the chronic muscular issues that lead to the problem in the first place. And, as you read in the pelvic tilt section, there can be a couple of different causes—tight hip flexors from too much sitting, weak abdominals, or even just lack of postural knowledge—all of which are dealt with extensively in these lessons.

---

23. I. A. Kapandji, (2008). *The Physiology of the Joints* (6th ed.). Edinburgh: Churchill Livingstone/Elsevier.

Excessive Lumbar Flexing

This particular point is fundamental to this manual and is mentioned, in one way or another, many times in these pages. However, it deserves to be specifically highlighted in this section and it is simply the notion that too much flexing of the lower back is bad for you.

In his article, "Spine flexion exercise: Myths, Truths and Issues affecting health and performance," Dr. Stuart McGill explains that:

> "Flexion movement of the spine strains the layers of collagen (connective and protective tissue) in the spinal discs... slowly the nucleus of the disc will work through... and create a disc bulge."[24]

This essentially means that with repetitive lumbar flexing (forward bending of the spine), repetitive stresses occur that lead to the micro traumas mentioned earlier. If the loads are light and the back is stabilized, the movement is healthy for the most part. But add more load, repeat or hold that posture for an extended period, and you could be in for significant long-term damage.

Get into a Standing Posture

Now that you have a deeper understanding of how

---

24 Stuart McGill. *Spine flexion exercise: Myths, Truths and Issues affecting health and performance*. Retrieved from Backfitpro. com: http://www.backfitpro.com/documents/Spine-flexion-myths-truths-and-issues.pdf

proper posture can help you, let's establish a good standing posture.

- Start with a firm base of support from your feet, feeling the whole foot attach to the ground. Remove your shoes so you can really experience the weight of your body evenly distributed across your feet.

- Make sure your feet are hip to shoulder-width apart, toes pointed straight ahead or just barely pointed outward, and that your knees are aligned over your toes.

- Make sure your knees are not locked. Unlocking your knees will allow them to correctly line up above the arches of your feet.

- Now slightly activate your abdominals and glutes to hold your pelvis in the neutral position (i.e. not in an anterior or posterior tilt).

- Draw your shoulders back and down, known as "packing" your shoulders.

- Allow your chest to lift up, or "puff out," just a bit and keep your eyes focused forward. "Chest out, eyes out" is a good way of thinking about this.

- Keep your chin level and lengthen yourself towards the ceiling as though there is a string pulling the top of your head straight up.

You will have created a straight line that goes from

your ankles, to just behind your knees, up through your shoulders, through the ear holes, and up past the top of your head. Depending on your baseline condition, you might also notice that certain muscles of the back and abs fatigue and become sore quickly. This is natural at first, because some of these muscles haven't been used correctly, if at all.

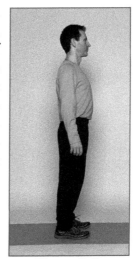

Figure 3-2
Good Posture

Go ahead and rest if you need to, but come right back to this proper posture and keep coming back to it. If you practice this correct posture, it will have the effect of "working out" the core muscles and strengthening the support for your lower back and hips.

The American Council on Exercise makes the point clearly that:

> "If the lumbar spine is correctly aligned with regard to the pelvis, and the pelvis is properly balanced in relation to the legs, the forces applied to the low-back can be reduced. Achieving this balance requires excellent muscular strength and flexibility..."[25]

I want to stress here that achieving better posture consistently, without thinking about it, does NOT happen

25. American Council on Exercise, op. cit.

overnight. I believe that improved posture and its resulting benefits are critical to healthy movement and a healthy lower back. Good posture may in fact be a "magic pill" for minimizing low-back pain, but it's a pill that you need to take every day.

Sitting Posture

Let me start this section by saying we should all do as little sitting as possible. Many studies have shown that too much sitting is related to increased risk of cardiovascular disease and cancer.[26] For our purposes, however, I'm just going to focus on some of the postural issues of sitting and what a "pain in the back" it can be.

I've mentioned what prolonged sitting can do to your hip flexors, but I want to explain it in a little more detail. As you now know, the hip flexors connect from the lumbar spine and front of the pelvis and attach to the upper part of your femur (thigh bone). When you sit, this muscle shortens. If you sit for extended periods without taking breaks to stand, in a way they will start to "believe" that the smaller length is the norm and will then allow themselves to degenerate to fit that norm.[27]

Of course, even though you're sitting for much of the day, you still need that muscle to extend when you stand.

26. David W. Dunstan, Alicia A. Thorp, and Genevieve N. Healy. "Prolonged Sitting." *Current Opinion in Cardiology* 26.5 (2011): 412-19. Web.

27. Sue E. Huether and Kathryn L. McCance, (2004). *Understanding Pathophysiology* (3rd edition). St. Louis, MO: Mosby.

A chronically shortened muscle doesn't want to extend and gives an unwanted tug instead. This will create havoc in the lower back and is a very common cause of significant back pain and back attacks. One of those reflex mechanisms I mentioned earlier is generally responsible for this effect: it senses a dangerous "pull," even though the muscle is really just extending back to its resting length to allow you to stand up.

But that's not the worst of it. The pressures on your discs can increase up to 40% when sitting, compared to standing.[28] So often coupled with a rounded lower back or shoulders that develops when we sit, it's a recipe for spinal trouble.

Keeping all of this in mind, it's easy to see the importance of a good sitting posture, not to mention regularly getting up and moving around. Finding an efficient sitting posture is very similar to doing it while standing.

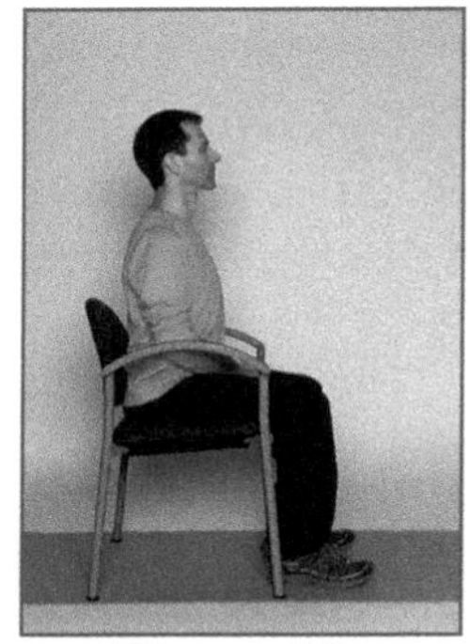

- Find your neutral spine, just as you did while standing, and make sure you draw your shoulders down and back (pack your shoulders).

- Imagine the string pulling from the top of your head to elongate your spine.

Figure 3-3

28. A. Nachemson. (1981). Disc pressure measurements. *Spine, 6* (1), 93-97.

- Make sure you maintain the three natural curves of your back. (Figure 3-3) Although you should always use your muscles to support your posture whenever possible, this is a good time to make use of a lumbar support, if needed.

- Try to only use a lumbar support to give your muscles time to rest from their new workload. Go back to relying on your muscles as soon as you can. Remember that an artificially-supported muscle will weaken over time.

- Continually check to make sure you're sitting squarely on both "cheeks."

- Ideally, your hips and knees should form a 90-degree angle to their adjoining parts, as shown in figure 3-3

- Try to avoid seats that dip down or sink in when you sit, as this design forces an unhealthy lumbar and sacral curve. A fold-up beach chair is an extreme example of this. Because of the sagging, unsupported nature of the seat bottom, it is a bad choice if you have low-back trouble...and, frankly, even if you don't.

- Avoid sitting in the same position for more than 30 minutes at a time and do everything you can to stand for at least 10 minutes each hour. The more healthy standing you can do, the better.

When it comes to sitting, it's important to remember that variation is the key. The posture I've described is a good one, but the best posture is the one that is always changing. The best chair to use is one that allows for adjustability. As Dr. McGill states in his book, *Low Back Disorders*:

> "Tissue loads must be migrated from tissue to tissue to minimize the risk of any single tissue accumulating micro trauma. This is accomplished by changing postures... the primary recommendation is to continually change the settings on the chair."[29]

As long as you make sure that you're not slouching, you should adjust your position regularly. This can include reclining, having feet on a foot rest, or even sitting cross-legged for a bit. Lean back and put the keyboard on your lap for ten minutes and, of course, get up as often as possible. As I type this, I am on my feet with the computer elevated. I'll sit again at some point, but won't stay that way for very long.

I want to stress again that if you have low-back troubles, then spending any amount of time in a soft, cushiony couch or lounge chair can be hazardous to your skeletal and muscular health. The surfaces you sit on should be firm enough for you to maintain proper posture. The softer the surface, the harder it is to keep your back straight

---

29.   Stuart McGill. (2007). *Low Back Disorders: Evidence-based Prevention and Rehabilitation.* (Second Edition.) Champaign, IL: Human Kinetics.

and supported. Not impossible, but much harder. If your muscles can "collapse" into a heap of stuffing and pillows, your spine will want to conform to whatever shape is created by that environment. This will inevitably lead to a rounded lower back, very shortened hip flexors and a high chance of low-back pain.

To protect your back even more, try not to twist your torso to get a file or hand something to a neighbor. Get up and out of the chair and stand or kneel in front of the file cabinet. And, of course, even one or two steps to the next cubicle is something your body will appreciate very much.

Spending a Lot of Time Driving

I've made this a separate section because I know that many people experience low-back discomfort from being in a car—sometimes for short drives, but more often after long distances or from having a job that requires you to be in a vehicle for extended periods of time. However, the simple fact is that everything I've described about a "sitting posture" also applies to being in a vehicle.

You may not be able to get up and walk around the car while driving, but you can stop and get out for a few minutes each hour on long trips. You can also use the various seat adjustments to slightly alter your position now and then. Of course, you want to maintain the spine's natural curves (neutral spine) and use the lumbar support if needed, but you also have the added ability to adjust the seat's back to recline more or less, or to move the entire seat back, forward, up or down. These slight changes in position can give your muscles a chance to move, even just a little, and prevent you from being in a static posture for too long.

While keeping your lower back supported, shoulders packed and eyes on the road, you can make use of whatever small adjustments your car offers to keep your posture varied and minimize the stiffness you'll experience from spending time on the road.

Lesson 4. Moving Smarter with Positional Postures

Although most of us think about standing or sitting up straight when we hear the word "posture," the Merriam-Webster Dictionary defines it as: "the position or bearing of the body, whether characteristic or assumed for a special purpose." Basically, the word applies to any physical position your body is in at a given moment, and throughout a given movement, i.e. bending, lifting, twisting, etc. And in every one of those "moments," it is crucial to be aware of, and to attend to, what I call your "positional posture."

In other words, practicing the best way to hold or move through a positional posture (which includes an awareness of core activation) will give you a great advantage in the fight against low-back pain. No matter what stationary posture (repairing a sink, watching a movie, or working at the computer) or moving posture (shifting furniture, reaching for a dish, or picking up a child) is involved, the need to pay attention and keep your "positional posture" strong and supported cannot be overstated.

And to be perfectly clear, a lot of what is discussed in *this* lesson requires a certain level of strength and balance that you will gain from following the actions in lesson five. So, if you find some of the techniques that are listed below a little more difficult than the old, inefficient and back-straining ways, don't lose hope. A strong and more vibrant life of healthy movement is within your reach.

Biomechanics vs. Ergonomics

This manual doesn't discuss "ergonomics," a term whose definition is often confused with "biomechanics." Essentially, ergonomics is the study of how the environment affects our postures and the process of changing that environment to better fit the way our bodies need to work. It definitely plays an important role in preventing repetitive micro traumas at work and in the home. Common ergonomics discussions involve how your office space is designed, how the utensils are set up around your kitchen, or simply making sure an emergency responder has the best tools to work with victims.

On the other hand, biomechanics studies how the body responds to, and moves against, the environment, whether it's ergonomically designed or not. You may have the best desk chair, set at the right height and angle, but how do you maintain the correct sitting posture while working at the desk all day? Your kitchen might be set up well, but you'll still have to bend down correctly to get into a lower cabinet. And, certainly, a first responder can't control the condition of a home or car when he or she arrives at the scene to give help. The positional postures discussed below will teach you how to maintain strength, stability and safety, using your body the way it was designed to be used, regardless of the ergonomics.

How to Lean Forward

A positional posture (and general movement) tip that is important to emphasize up front is simply about how to lean forward. Although many back injuries occur while lifting, contorting for some task or another, or even just twisting incorrectly, a considerable strain is placed on your back muscles and spine when you simply lean over to shave, do the dishes, or just to reach for something beyond arm's length.

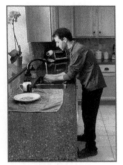 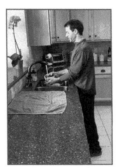 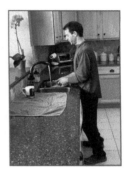

Figure 4-1   Figure 4-2   Figure 4-3

As I mentioned in the section on "bad postures," continuous bending of the spine, even with the relatively light load of just your upper body, can lead to damage. Remember that the torso can be 65% or more of our body weight and, as soon as you tilt the torso away from its center so it's no longer over the hips, you place added strain on the structures trying to hold you upright, increasing the stress by over 100%.[30]

It is especially important to activate the core when leaning forward. I've made this point previously, but understanding this simple concept is a big part of many of the following positional postures. As with the posture shown in Figure 4-1, for example, you may round your

---

30. A. Nachemson, op. cit.

back when you reach over a sink to do dishes. You can see in the other two sink pictures, however, that I'm keeping my spine neutral.

Contract the abs, especially the TVA, and hold them strongly until your torso is back above your lower body. If you've got too much belly and need to lean farther to reach the sink, you might find that bracing your knees against the cabinet below (if there is one available) will add support to the posture. Either way, the moment you lean forward is the moment an abdominal and core exercise should begin.

If you need to "crawl" into the back of your SUV or work vehicle, make sure you're stabilizing your spine as you make the transition from standing to being "on all fours." Even more importantly, if you spend extended time inside a cargo area that's lower than your height, like ambulance or postal workers do, you must maintain an active core at all times while "hunched over." The more often you're hunched over in that environment, the greater your chance for disc problems. Following these lessons helps keep those problems at bay for as long as possible.

The Right Way to Lower and Lift

Many people have heard "lift with your legs, not your back," as that's probably the most commonly expressed way to keep your back safe, but more direction is definitely needed. What's often left out is the question of *how* you "bend down" in the first place. When I say "bend down," I don't mean "bend over," as I discussed above. What I am talking about is how to get to the floor or into a lower position to tie your shoe or pick up something, and there are two basic techniques that work well for this.

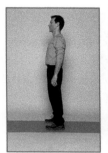 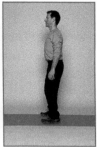 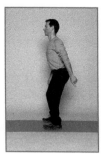 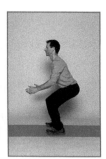

Figure 4-4   Figure 4-5   Figure 4-6   Figure 4-7

"Squat" Technique

- Start this movement with a slight anterior tilt of the pelvis and backwards hip thrust (imagine pouring water out of the pelvic "basin" over the front of your legs). A "squat" should not start through the legs or knees. (Figure 4-5)

- Continue driving your glutes/hips back as though you're about to sit in a chair, (Figure 4-6)

- Keep your spine neutral (Figures 4-4 through 4-7).

- Many people have heard that "your knees shouldn't go past your toes," but the truth is, as long as you're not *actively* sending your knees forward (i.e. leading the movement with your hips instead), it's okay if the knees go past the toes. For someone with long legs, it might be mechanically impossible to avoid.

- As you prepare to straighten up, make sure you feel your feet firmly against the ground.

- The effort for the lifting motion should start in your mid-foot and heels and, as you push against the ground, you'll be taking advantage of the strength from your upper legs, not your back. (This is where we get "lift with your legs, not your back.")

- As always, your core should continue to support your lower back. Do *not* adjust the curve of your spine *while* your back is actively supporting a lifting effort, as that can lead to serious issues.[31]

- As you straighten your body towards the top of the "lift," remember to fully elongate, straightening your legs and lengthening your torso above your hips in the same motion, and bring your pelvis back into neutral.

You also often hear "keep your back straight," when referring to proper lifting mechanics, but that phrase causes some misunderstanding. That direction simply means to make sure that your back is not "rounded." It does not mean you have to keep your back in a straight up and down position. In fact, unless your lower back and

31. Stuart McGill. *Spine flexion exercise: Myths, Truths and Issues affecting health and performance.* Retrieved from Backfitpro. com: http://www.backfitpro.com/documents/Spine-flexion-myths-truths-and-issues.pdf

ankles are very loose and flexible, keeping it straight up and down during a squatting movement is very difficult. Thankfully, it's also not necessary for a safe lift, as long as you keep your spine neutral and supported. Remembering "chest out (just a bit), eyes out" will help you to keep your back properly straight during this move.

Kneeling or "Lunging"

The other (and possibly far more useful) way of getting into a lower position is to kneel or (as it's called in the exercise world) lunge. All of us have knelt down many times in our lives, but most of us have missed the idea I mentioned above—keeping your back straight. I've already spoken at length about the idea of a straight and supported back, but now I want to incorporate it into this positional posture.

When you kneel, it's common to bend over more than you should Many of us don't even kneel fully to the ground, but just partially lower ourselves and bend the torso the rest of the way to pick up the object (Figure 4-8). This is a big mistake.

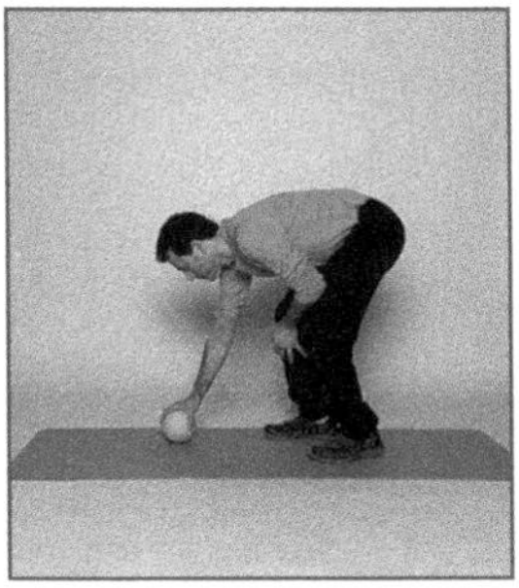

Figure 4-8

- Start from a good standing posture and step one foot forward, towards the object to be lifted.

- Keeping your upper body stabilized above the waist (sound familiar?), move your hips straight down towards the floor.

- Once you've grabbed the item from the floor, file drawer, or baby stroller, push up and slightly backwards through the mid-foot and heel of your forward leg, "driving" your body towards the back foot and into an upright position. (Figures 4-9 to 4-12).

- Stabilize yourself as you get fully straightened up and continue on with your day.

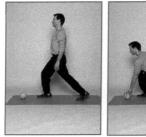 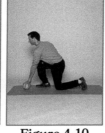 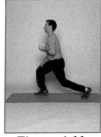 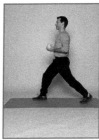

Figure 4-9   Figure 4-10   Figure 4-11   Figure 4-12

Twisting

A twisting back attack can seem to occur out of nowhere. This is largely because we neglect to activate our core prior to the movement. In other words, like with any other movement, twisting has to start, continue, and end with strong and stable support of your pelvis and lower back. Rotating the upper body without supporting the core leaves the surrounding muscles and joints susceptible to over-extensions, rapid tightening and spasm.

One of the reasons a simple twist needs so much muscular support is because of the structure of the lumbar spine. Along the entire spine, each vertebra is connected to the next by what's called a "facet joint." The alignment of this joint is one of the major limiting factors that determines how far, and in which direction, different parts of the spine can move.

In the lower back, the facet joints are aligned in such a way so as to greatly limit how far we can twist side to side. If we go too far (and that's not far at all!), the joint can "lock up" up and the rest of the motion is carried out through the disc itself.[32] Simply leaning and rotating at the same time can increase the load on the discs by more than a whopping 400%.[33]

The tiny muscles connecting each vertebra can sense this strain and will respond to the danger. A surprise to many is that this type of injury is not related to the amount of weight you are trying to carry or move; it is entirely about *proper* movement.

Making sure that your knees, toes and nose are all pointing in the same direction is another good way to stay safe during a twisting movement. Although this tip is mostly for keeping your knees healthy, it can also have an impact on your hips and lower back. Imagine wearing spikes on the bottom of your shoes that keep your feet stuck in place and then trying to move your body in a new direction. If your foot stays in place while the rest of your body is moving, you could easily injure any part of the muscle and joint chain from your feet to your back.

32. Phil Dodge, op. cit.
33. A. Nachemson, op. cit.

If you're moving something from one shelf or table to another, or simply turning to go in a different direction, be sure to point your foot and knee in that new direction while shifting your torso. Then, when ready, turn your face so your nose is lined up with your knee and toes and start moving.

Standing from a Sit

Many of us lean forward as we begin to stand from a seated position (Figure 4-13). This is a commonly recommended method for people who struggle with getting up and makes the movement feel easier. However, the reality is that this motion makes certain muscles work harder than they should to

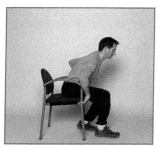

Figure 4-13

support the torso against gravity. Instead, following the same directions I've given about lifting and leaning, the safest way to stand from a chair is to keep your torso aligned above the waist as much as possible.

- Start by moving to the edge of the seat (Figure 4-14).

- Stabilize your back and, leading very slightly with your chest out, push up through the mid-foot and heels (Figures 4-15 and 4-16).

- Of course, you can use the arms or seat of the chair or other support to help you push yourself up, if needed.

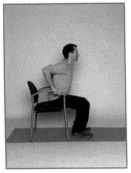 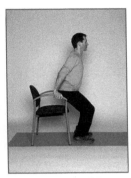 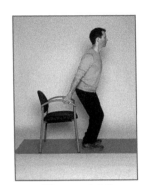

| Figure 4-14 | Figure 4-15 | Figure 4-16 |

You'll be using what strength you have in your upper legs, which will feel very different after a lifetime of using your back for momentum. As I've mentioned, your legs may not be ready for the task. Push off the chair with your hands (as shown), if needed, or use a wall or table to help with the move, but stop throwing your back into it.

Getting up from the Floor

As with many of the movement changes I'm giving you, the following technique for getting up from the floor may not seem natural. However, it is a simple, safe and effective way to move through this positional posture.

- From your position on the floor, start by aligning and lengthening your torso above your hips. Remember to keep your core active.

- Place a hand on the floor, a table or chair for support, and shift yourself into a kneeling position.

- • Push through the mid-foot and heel of the forward foot, just as described in the "kneeling or lunging" section.

A Good and Bad Night's Sleep

Your sleeping position is one of the least talked-about postures that affects back pain and your overall health. It's surprising that not more attention is paid to this concept, considering how much time we spend trying to get a good night's sleep. During this lesson, I'm not going to discuss the tremendous, positive value of sleep in our lives, but I do want to touch on how our sleeping postures can have such a significant impact on low-back pain.

Long-term muscle imbalances created by standing and seated postures can make things very uncomfortable when it's time to sleep. People with tight hip flexors may find it difficult to lie on their back, especially with their legs straight out. As the muscles and fascia tighten even more overnight, it can become more painful (and even dangerous) to get out of bed.

Unfortunately, sleeping on the side of your body or on your stomach can also create problems. Side-sleeping promotes rounding of the shoulders and often results in the bottom shoulder tucking under and in front of the torso, negatively affecting the shoulder and back.[34] Also, depending on the softness of the mattress, sleeping on your side allows your hips to dip out of alignment with the spine. A pillow between your knees will help alleviate

---

34. Justin Price (2009), op. cit.

some of that misalignment, and may lessen the morning pain.

Many of the people I speak to prefer to sleep on their stomach, although a good number of those folks admit that they experience some back pain in the morning. In fact, the people who are able to sleep this way *without pain* are usually younger, because they have not had their postural imbalances long enough to experience chronic pain from this position.

That being said, sleeping on your stomach will inevitably cause your lower back to arch excessively and, unless you're sleeping face down in the pillow, will also cause your neck to stay in a twisted position for an extended period of time. Anyone who has ever awakened with a sore muscle from "sleeping wrong" knows a little about what these postures can do to you.

For many people, as much as it feels "just not right" to sleep on their back, generally speaking, it is the best option. In time, once you get past the instinctive discomfort of being so "exposed" by sleeping in an open and unprotected position, you'll begin to feel much better when you wake up each morning. However, for folks with tight hip flexors, placing a pillow under your knees will lessen the strain on your lower back by disengaging those muscles.

I also hate to break it to so many of you out there, but your soft, plushy mattress might not be helping your back issues. If your mattress is too soft, it allows your body to lose the alignment you work so hard to achieve during the day; that's 6–8 hours of putting your muscles back into the wrong position. Your pillow should help support your head and neck to keep the cervical curve in place, as well.

As with all the new movements I describe in this manual, it will take practice to adjust your sleeping posture. Try to begin the night in a better position, coming back to it throughout the night if you wake up. Gradually, your body (and mind) will begin to adjust and you can spend a third of your life practicing good posture while you sleep.

The Morning Rise

When you suffer with nagging back pain for most of your waking hours, it's a great relief to wake up in the morning feeling good, even if it's only occasionally. However, that feeling of relief can be short-lived when you try to actually get out of bed and suddenly feel that jarring pain again.

While we sleep, our discs get some relief from the pressures of our daily lives and this gives them a chance to relax and rehydrate. That rehydration, however, occurs with fluids from our joints and this can make us feel stiff when we wake. Nonetheless, much of the discomfort of rising from bed can be avoided by following these easy guidelines to slowly and gently stretch before trying to raise your body.

- While lying flat on the bed, slide down toward the foot of the bed a bit, so there's room to raise your arms from your sides all the way over your head, to "reach" behind you. Try to feel a stretch in the torso. Feel your whole body lengthen for the duration of 4 or 5 breaths.

- Also, while on your back, gently bring your knees to your chest and hold that position for 4–5 breaths. You can keep your arms overhead, gently wrap them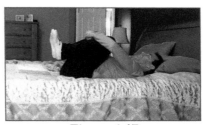

  Figure 4-17

  around your knees (Figure 4-17), or just leave them by your sides.

- Don't roll up too far into a ball during this move. Flex at the hip joint, not the waist, and keep your spine long and neutral.

At this point, you could do an arm-assisted sit-up—that is, do a full sit-up, but with your arms pushing on the bed behind you for assistance, raise your torso and then follow the instructions for "standing from a sit," as previously described (page 78). However, although it is a bit unusual, the method described below is much easier on your lower back.

- After your brief stretch, roll onto either side of your body and gently continue to roll over onto your stomach, while allowing your lower body to gently slide off the bed. This should put you in a kneeling position by the side of the bed.

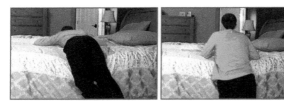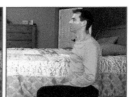

Figure 4-18   Figure 4-19   Figure 4-20

- From the kneeling position, get your torso in line with your hips and lift yourself up as was described for the lunge/kneeling position mentioned earlier.

The Power to Pull and Push

Have you ever tried to open a door that was heavier than you thought it was? The surprise tug on your arm, as well as on the rest of your body, can be very jarring. Whether opening a door, dragging a bag of autumn leaves across the yard, or retrieving equipment from the back of your vehicle, the power to pull must come from your active core. If you initiate the movement from a stable core while you create a wide, staggered base of support with your legs (Feet hip- or shoulder-width apart, with one foot in front of the other) and keep your shoulders down and back, then any load will be significantly easier to pull around.

Even though you can improve your ability to pull, it's always a better idea to push, if possible. A good pull technique can go a long way, but it doesn't make use of the added strength of the rest of your body that pushing does. By creating a good base with your legs, maintaining an active core, and keeping your hands at chest height when possible, your entire weight can be harnessed to push everything—from a piece of furniture to a car that is stuck in snow or mud.

Regardless of the choice to pull, push, twist, lift or lean, each and every positional posture must start and end with the core. It should be more than clear that everything you do during the course of work, life and play can be made stronger and safer with an effectively-stabilized lower back. In order to maintain that stability and keep your muscles in the balanced condition I've been talking about, let's get to the final lesson of the manual and go through some key actions to achieve and maintain that healthy balance.

Lesson 5: Achieving Muscle Balance

Now that I've taught you how your back, pelvis and hip area are designed by nature to support and stabilize movement, why this area can cause so much trouble, and how to move through life with more strength and confidence, you have a great foundation to stay strong and pain-minimized, but one more lesson is needed in this fight against low-back pain.

What you've learned so far will go a long way, but without achieving effective, long-term muscle balance and stability, you'll continue to be physically limited. This final lesson teaches you the valuable techniques and exercises that increase your advantage against back pain and give you the strength for years of active living.

Precautions

Before we get into it, though, there are some important precautions I want you to keep in mind if you've been diagnosed with an underlying skeletal problem, such as a disc issue, arthritis, stenosis, spondylolisthesis or other back condition.

Flexing your spine (bending forward) tends to create space in the spinal column, which reduces pressure on the nerves and can alleviate the symptoms of arthritis or stenosis,[35] both of which create a narrowing in the spinal column. On the other hand, bending backward (extending your spine) can create additional compression and possibly worsen the symptoms.[36]

The opposite is important for disc issues, many of which involve the vertebra's discs protruding out through the back of the spine from too much unsupported flexing. Think of bending two ends of a stick towards each other: the pressure builds in the middle until BAM! The middle gives in and bursts apart. Over time, this can happen to our discs. In this case, continuing to flex forward would aggravate the situation. Instead, arching or extending your back would create space and pressure to potentially allow the disc to "re-set" itself.[37,38]

Someone with spondylolisthesis, a condition where a vertebra shifts forward over the one below it, might be safer if they avoid both flexing and extending exercises. Instead, they might gain strength from isometric actions (causing a muscle to contract while neither lengthening

---

35. David Joseph Ponte, MA, PT, Gail J. Jensen, MA, PT and Barbara E. Kent, MA, PT (1984, Sep/Oct). A preliminary report on the use of the McKenzie protocol versus Williams protocol in the treatment of low back pain. *Journal of Orthopaedic & Sports Physical Therapy*, 130-139.
36. Phil Dodge, op. cit.
37. M. A. Adams, S. May, B. J. Freeman, H. P. Morrison, and P. Dolan, (2000). Effects of backward bending on lumbar intervertebral discs. Relevance to physical therapy treatments for low back pain. *Spine, 25* (4), 431-437.
38. Phil Dodge, op. cit.

nor shortening, but while remaining at a single length).[39] Anytime you hold yourself still and upright, you are experiencing isometric contractions.

Remember, though, that each back issue is unique, and I am not specifically recommending a particular exercise for any particular spinal disorder. I am simply trying to help you understand how to use your body and muscles to finally take control of your low-back pain. Please, take these next actions with caution and consult your doctor before starting any exercise program.

Anatomy Re-Cap

I've already made it clear how your effort to maintain the natural curves of the spine can have a significant impact on your low-back health, so I won't cover that again. However, I do want to reiterate the value of the joint that connects the upper and lower parts of our bodies— the SI joint. Since our ability to move smoothly and with stability is partially dependent on this joint, as we transfer the physical forces between the two halves of the body, the care and maintenance of the muscles surrounding it is very important.

There are a large number of muscles in this area but, for the sake of this lesson, we'll continue to focus on the four main muscle groups we've been discussing throughout the manual. Although we can't avoid the micro traumas in our tissues, or easily control the response of the smaller spinal

---

39. Stuart McGill. (2007). *Low Back Disorders: Evidence-based Prevention and Rehabilitation.* (Second Edition.) Champaign, IL: Human Kinetics.

muscles to the dangers of poor mechanics, these larger muscles are ones that we can affect. Managing these muscle groups effectively can have a tremendous, positive impact on our low-back pain.

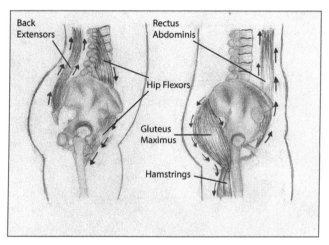

Figure 5-1: Pelvic Tilt, showing the direction of pull from the key muscle groups

By keeping the pelvic tilt image in mind, you can remember the various relationships that the key muscles have with each other.

The abdominal muscles work cooperatively with the hamstrings and the glutes to tilt the pelvis back, causing the hip joint to move forward and reducing (flattening) the lumbar curve.

At the same time, the back extensors and hip flexors work together to create an anterior (forward) pelvis tilt, driving the hip joint backwards, which results in an increase in the lumbar curve. It's important to point out, as well, that all four of these groups work together by counteracting each other to hold the pelvis in a neutral position (not tilted in either direction).

While these muscles are working to control pelvic tilt, the left or right side of the body can be (and often is) dominant over the other. This imbalance can cause a subtle but very unwanted twist at the SI joint, which can result in a "protective" reaction in even the smallest muscles, and very likely lead to some level of pain and possibly a disabling "back attack."

Key Actions

There are several actions you can take to revitalize, balance and strengthen your muscles over the long-term. This manual is not specifically about stretching, self-massage or strength training, and so it will not provide extensive education in these areas.

If you have the opportunity, I highly recommend that you find a good chiropractor and massage therapist. Muscle imbalance from a lifetime of poor mechanics and incessant gravity can pull your spine, shoulders and hips out of alignment. A quality chiropractor can readjust your skeleton to give those muscles "space" and time to get back into balance. (However, if you don't do your share of the muscle work, as described in this manual, this benefit is lost.) I also strongly advocate self-massage, but if you have access to a licensed massage therapist, I suggest that you include that service in your regimen, as well.

The following instructions and precautions will give you a good foundation of three key actions: 1) self-myofascial release (I also use the term "self-massage"); 2) stretching; and 3) strength work. Explore these further with your doctor, an exercise specialist, physical or massage therapist or personal trainer, and spend the time to learn what works best for you.

- For the best results, always do fascia release first, stretch next, and then strengthen.

- Always exhale on the more difficult part of exercise (i.e. during the exertion), and inhale on the relaxation. Breathe deeply into your lungs and use your core (including your diaphragm) to stabilize the spine and give you strength while you exhale.

- In any instance where I've offered more than one massage, stretch, or strengthen for a particular muscle, you only need to choose one.

- The exceptions to the previous rule are crunches and planks. They are both listed as strength actions for the abs but the plank focuses much more work on the TVA, whereas crunches provide more work for the rectus abdominis and obliques. Both of these exercises should be done.

- To ensure correct form, perform these actions with a partner who has read through this manual, if possible. A mirror will also be helpful to identify needed adjustments.

- Unless otherwise directed, always try to work on a mat or carpet. Avoid hard floors if possible, especially when your knees are on the ground.

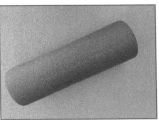

- Make sure you include a chair or other appropriately stable support.

Figure 5-2
Foam Roller

Self-Myofascial Release

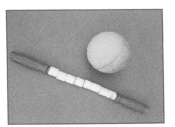

The fascia tissue in our bodies not only connects all the internal muscles and organs of the body, it also helps control movement and conveys information about our balance, position and overall internal health. Because of the fascia's critical role in movement and well-being, deeply massaging and "releasing" the tissue when it's tightened or bound up is an important step in managing muscle pain and movement health.[40]

Figure 5-3
Massage Ball, "Stick"

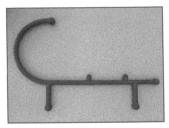

Figure 5-4
Thera Cane

Deep self-massage (myofascial release) realigns and rejuvenates the tissue and muscles. This can bring immediate relief of symptoms and provides a more receptive environment for stretching and strengthening.

---

40. Justin Price (2009), op. cit.

Using your hands can work for certain muscles, but I strongly encourage you to invest a few dollars in a foam roller, a tennis or massage ball, and a "stick" or Thera Cane (Figures 5-2, 5-3 and 5-4). All of these can be found on Amazon.com, at your local sporting goods stores, or even in larger supermarkets, for as little as $5. These tools will allow for a much deeper fascia release than you can achieve with your hands.

- Never do fascia release over a torn muscle or tendon until it has healed sufficiently. Gentle—not deep— massage may be appropriate to improve blood flow and assist healing, but your doctor should advise you on this.

- As you apply pressure you will very likely feel some painful spots. You should focus on these spots; the instructions for addressing those points are described in the abdominal fascia release section.

- I need to be very clear that when you release tight fascia and muscles in this way, you will experience a certain level of discomfort or pain, especially at those painful spots. In fact, the closer you are to a flare-up, the more painful these spots could be. Your tolerance for this pain is the only limiting factor.

- Some of the techniques require a certain level of balance or stamina, and can be a bit of a strength workout on their own. If one method is too difficult, then another one may work for you.

- Unless otherwise noted, fascia release exercises can be just 1-2 minutes in duration, depending on your tolerance and stamina. In an ideal world, they should be done daily.

Stretching

This key action helps improve mobility, flexibility and stability. It also improves muscle efficiency after long-term poor posture and inappropriate movement.[41] Although there are many different types of stretching, this lesson covers only what is useful for our purpose. I'll also highlight what you need to know to do these stretches safely and effectively.

A good general rule is to avoid stretching a muscle that is in use, because a muscle under tension is much harder to stretch. For example, this is why you are instructed to do the "standing quad stretch" with support. During that action, the quad you're trying to stretch will be activated to help keep you balanced and upright and will resist the stretch. Putting as much of your weight as you can on the support and on the non-stretched leg allows the quad to "disengage," and makes this stretch much more effective and safe.

Please keep in mind that a relaxed muscle also needs to be strengthened, creating just the right muscle "tone" (not either "hypertonic" or "hypotonic," as described in

41. Arnold G. Nelson and Jouko Kokkonen. (2007). *Stretching anatomy*. Champaign, IL: Human Kinetics.

the first lesson). When you stretch, you are essentially "loosening" the stability at the joint, which results in a desirable increase in its range of motion. However, if that muscle isn't also strengthened, there is an increased likelihood of over-extending that joint. In other words, joint stability depends on both: muscle balance and tone.

- Hold a stretch for as long as it takes to feel the stretch release. That is, as you get into a particular stretch position, you'll move your body as instructed until you begin to feel the first sense of tightness. That's where you stop moving, hold the stretch, and continue to breathe deeply until the tension releases. This is where the "hold a stretch for 20–30 seconds" comes from. It may take that much time for the tension to release, but it's important to learn to *feel it* for yourself, instead of relying on a timer, so you can get a more effective stretch.

- Once you feel the tension *release* within the muscle, then—and only then—you can stretch that muscle a little further until you reach the next sense of tightness. Hold the stretch again (without moving further) until the tightness releases. Then move on to stretch another muscle.

- If you remember the two reflex mechanisms that I mentioned in the "muscle in action" section of the Anatomy lesson, then you know why you can't force or push through a stretch; the muscles are designed to push back. In fact, the release of tension you feel while you are stretching is not just the muscle fibers' response; it is also the relaxation of the stretch reflex.

- Be patient and breathe. You can increase the effect of a stretch by imagining your breath going directly into the area being worked on. This is why therapists will often instruct their clients to "breathe into" the area they are working on. It promotes overall relaxation, and focusing your attention on a given area is a very powerful tool for improving a particular condition.

- In an ideal world, where you're strengthening and massaging regularly, you should stretch a little bit every day.

- As with myofascial release, do not stretch the area of a recently torn muscle or tendon.

Strengthening

This section is not about building big muscles, or even achieving a better-looking body. The strengthening work you'll learn is specifically intended to build overall stability within your core, which will result in increased overall endurance and stronger, pain-minimized living.

I want to mention the importance of pacing during many of these strengthening actions. Adjusting the pace of a given exercise helps to ensure that you're getting the most effective workout. You can alter how difficult it is to do an exercise simply by speeding up or slowing down the movement. This is one of the reasons that using only your body weight works so well. As you've learned throughout this manual, your body is constantly working against gravity. Eventually, this should feel effortless in daily life, but for many of us, it's strenuous enough to be a good workout. That means you probably carry around enough natural body weight to do strengthening work wherever you are.

Being able to adjust how the weight of your body feels is also a valuable benefit. For example, if you *decrease* how quickly you move your leg up and down, you *increase* how much time those muscles have to work against gravity. This increases the workload and effort needed and makes your leg feel "heavier." If you speed up the motion, you decrease the work and effort needed and it feels easier. Kids know this intuitively, and it's why they move quickly across monkey bars. If they pause or move more slowly, it increases the stress to the muscles and makes it much more difficult for them to get to the other side.

Keep in mind that, if you move too quickly through a set of leg lifts—literally throwing your leg up and down— it gives very little benefit. It is more likely that it will hurt you, because speed usually means less control, and a greater potential for injury. No matter what pace you feel comfortable with, always make sure you're in control of your movements and using the best mechanics possible.

For our purposes of being safe and building muscle endurance, a count of two in each direction is a good place to start. As you gain strength and proficiency, you can "advance" to a slower pace, just as someone might add weight to a barbell. This ability to adjust the effort makes these body weight exercises very flexible. Continue to adjust your pacing and you'll always be challenged.

- There are certain strengthening actions where breathing can be difficult and potentially dangerous. This would be during an action that requires you to hold a position, i.e. perform an isometric or static muscle contraction (the plank, for example). While you are in these types of positions, the muscles that enable you to breathe are busy holding you in that position, so they may not be available to work the lungs. I have noted where it may be appropriate to briefly hold your breath. You can also breathe through pursed lips (inhale through your nose and exhale through pursed lips), as this will isolate the diaphragm better and make breathing easier and safer during those types of movements.

- It may go without saying, but these strengthening exercises are not to be done if you're experiencing an actual back attack. If a strength exercise hurts, don't do it. Stick with fascia release and stretch until you can do the strength work without pain.

- All of the strength exercises described in this manual can be done every day, but should be done *no less than* three times a week.

- Rest for at least one or two minutes between sets of any given exercise, unless otherwise noted.

Abdominals

Fascia Release

You've probably never seen someone massaging his or her abs but it can make a huge difference in controlling your low-back pain. In fact, I've discovered that this action is most useful when your pain level is high, such as right after or during an actual back attack. Some folks feel very little from this action when pain is low.

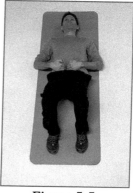

Figure 5-5
Fascia Release

- Lie on your back with feet flat on the floor and knees up, or just place a pillow under your knees. Keeping your legs bent helps deactivate the hip flexors and keep your pelvis neutral.

- Using three or four fingers, gently (but firmly) begin applying downward pressure into the belly. Apply pressure all around the area, from just above the belly button, out to the sides by your ribs, and down below the pelvic bone.

- Once you find a tender spot, or spots, take a deep breath and, while you exhale, press down and hold for a count of seven; release for a count of three while you inhale. Don't worry too much about getting this count exactly right. Just try to apply some pressure during an exhale and release the pressure on the inhale. Do three sets of compression/release and then move to another spot.

- Depending on what condition your back is in at the time, this can be painful. The worse your back pain, the worse the abdominal tender spots will feel, so continue to breathe deeply and know that you're on your way to making a big difference.

Stretch

Abdominal stretching is not one of the easier stretches to do, but give it try—slowly. As with all the movement practices, if you do it often enough, you'll get better and more effective.

Cobra

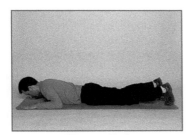
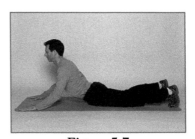

Figure 5-6   Figure 5-7

- Lie on your belly with your palms and forearms on the ground, as shown in Figure 5-6.

- Gently push your shoulders and torso up with the arms. Extend only as far as is comfortable.

- Keep your pelvis on the ground, your neck straight, and always be lengthening the spine, as though a string is pulling from the top of your head

- If you're able to feel a stretch, hold it until it releases, and if you have the strength, try and extend a little further into a second stretch.

- This can be a difficult movement, so if it isn't working for you, don't worry. Just move on.

Standing Abdominal Stretch

- Stand upright, in good posture.

- Raise your arms overhead, reaching slightly backward into an extension behind the line of your body.

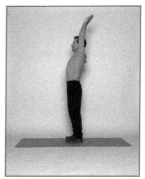

- If you need to limit the degree of extension, try reaching straight up or stretch your arms over your head while lying on your back.

Figure 5-8
Standing Abdominal
Stretch

- Reach towards the ceiling, lengthening your torso while you slightly and gently lift the chest up and outward.

- Allow your back to arch slightly, but always be lengthening it at the same time.

- To focus more on the obliques, add a slight side bend.

Strength

Crunch

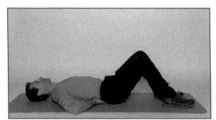 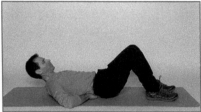

| Figure 5-9 | Figure 5-10 |

Mostly works the rectus abdominis and obliques.

- Start on your back with your knees bent, feet flat on the ground, arms down by your sides. DO NOT flatten your back against the floor, as many people suggest. If needed, support the curve of your lower back with your hands, as shown in Figures 5-9 and 5-10.

- Maintain the cervical curve. It might help to press your tongue against the roof of your mouth just behind your teeth. This engages the muscles that stabilize your neck.

- Take a breath and exhale while slightly "curling" your shoulders and chest towards your belly button until you feel the work in your abs.

- You might only need to lift your shoulders and chest a few inches from the ground to feel an effective activation of the abs.

- You should NOT bring your chest all the way up to your knees, as this activates the hip flexors and can potentially pull the lumbar spine into hyperextension, which will cause significant stress and pain in the lower back.

- Inhale and slowly—*with control*—lower yourself back to the ground.

- Work towards two sets of 12 reps.

- To focus on your obliques, add a very slight twist, alternating towards one knee and then the other.

- Focus on your obliques for one of the two sets.

Plank

This will work many muscles throughout the body, but is primarily useful for the deeper stabilizing muscles of the abs, specifically the TVA.

- This is an action where breathing through pursed lips is recommended.

- Lie on your stomach with forearms on the ground, elbows tucked in to your sides and directly under your shoulders. Your hands can be flat on floor or

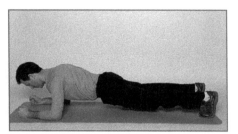

Figure 5-11, Plank

clenched into fists. Clasping your hands together can offer a little extra support for this move.

- Straighten your legs, and tuck your toes towards your shins.

- Activate your abs and TVA and slowly lift yourself off of the floor, keeping your whole body in a strong, straight line from your heels to the tip of your head.

- Leg muscles and glutes should be tensed.

- Do not allow your hips, lower back or ribs to sag at all. Your body must remain strong throughout the entire exercise.

- Try not to lift your hips into the air or bend your knees for any added support.

- No shrugging or bringing your shoulders up towards your ears.

- Keep the core strong and your body in a straight

line, from your heels to the top of your head. Hold this position for 10–20 seconds.

- Slowly—*with control*—lower yourself back to the floor, knees first.

- Rest for a minute or so and try once more.

- The goal is to eventually hold this position for up to 60 seconds. For now, only hold it until you feel your lower back muscles fatiguing. Do not let those muscles "collapse." Make sure you are in control of the movement at all times.

Hip Flexors—Iliacus and Psoas

Since the hip flexors are chronically tight in so many of us, fascia release and stretching should be the main focus. The first action in the list is very similar to the abdominal fascia release.

Fascia Release

- Lie on your back with your knees bent upward and your feet flat on the ground. Keep your pelvis neutral.

- Using three or four fingers, gently begin applying downward pressure into the lower part of the belly, about 2 inches to the side of and an inch or so lower than the belly button (Figure 5-12).

- If you slowly raise and lower one knee towards your

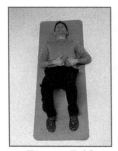
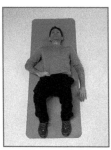
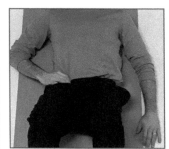

Figure 5-12
Psoas release

Figure 5-13
Iliacus release

Figure 5-13
Iliacus release, closeup

chest, you might be able to feel the psoas working. This will help you to better locate the muscle.

- For the iliacus, you'll need to move the work to the side of the pelvis along the top edge of the hip (Figures 5-13 and 14). There's a chance this area is very sensitive to pressure so take it slow and easy.

- Refer to Figure 5-14, as well as the "Hip Flexors" section of the Anatomy lesson (page 41) for more details on locations.

- Address tender points, as explained in the abdominal fascia release section.

- Depending on the condition of your back, this can be painful, so continue to breathe deeply and keep going.

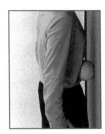

- This action can also be achieved by using a tennis or massage ball against a wall. (Figure 5-15)

Figure 5-15

- Stand facing a sturdy wall and place the ball between you and the wall at the location of the tender spot on the muscle. Make sure there are no switches, plugs or artwork on the wall where you're working.

- Move your body around while pressing against the ball. This will require some work from your legs as you use your body to maneuver around the wall and adjust the pressure, as needed.

- Stop and address tender spots as you find them.

Stretch

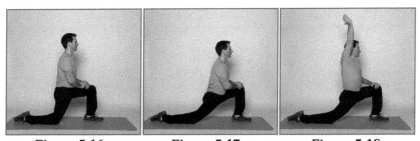

Figure 5-16   Figure 5-17   Figure 5-18

Lunge Stretch

- Get into a kneeling position with your left foot forward. Make sure your left knee is placed over your ankle, and your left hip is bent to about 90 degrees, with your thigh parallel to the floor. (Figure 5-16).

- Make sure your torso is lengthened and aligned above your pelvis with a supported, neutral spine.

- Press forward and down with your hips while keeping your right knee pressed into the ground (Figure 5-17).

- Stop when you begin to feel the stretch on your right side and hold until the stretch releases.

- If desired, lunge a little deeper to feel a second stretch. Hold until it releases; then switch legs and repeat.

- Do not allow your pelvis to tilt forward or one hip to shift higher or lower than the other.

- If you need to, use a wall, chair, etc. for support and balance.

To further isolate the psoas, raise your arm (on the stretched side) over your head, reaching towards the opposite side (Figure 5-18).

Strength

Lying-Straight Leg Raise

Strengthening these muscles is challenging for people with low-back issues because the movement needed can tug on the lumbar spine. Please follow the directions below and do this exercise very carefully. Placing your hands or arms under your lower back is a good way to help support neutral stability during this movement (Figure 5-19).

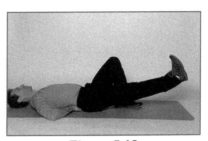

Figure 5-19
Lying-Straight Leg Raise

- Lie on your back with one leg straight out and the other bent with your foot flat on the floor.

- Activate your core to stabilize a neutral pelvis and spine.

- With control, lift the straight leg up a few inches and then return it to the floor.

- Keep your leg straight throughout movement and the toes of that foot pointed up.

- If you feel your lower back straining from this movement, stop the exercise and avoid it until your abdominals are strong enough to provide the necessary support.

- Do not speed through this or quickly "pump" the

leg up and down. Use a slow count of two in each direction.

- Work towards two sets of 12 reps for each leg.

Hip Flexor—Rectus Femoris

Fascia release

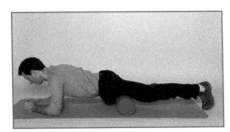

Figure 5-20

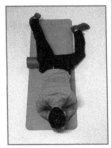

Figure 5-21

- Place a foam roller perpendicular to the leg you are going to work on and lie over it, putting pressure on your thigh (Figure 5-20).

- Use your arms and the opposite leg for support and to help manipulate your body over the roller (Figure 5-21).

- Maneuver yourself forward and back along the roller, and locate tender points.

- Feel free to rotate your body while you roll backward and forward to release fascia on the rest of the thigh, but be careful when you get to the outside of the thigh (iliotibial band), because this area can be very tender and painful in many people.

- Do not roll directly over the kneecap.

- This action can be done on a single leg or both legs simultaneously.

- Roll back and forth for 1–2 minutes on each leg; then move on.

A massage stick is also an effective option if you're unable to use the foam roller as described.

Sit comfortably on the floor or a chair.

- Relax one of your legs by slightly bending the knee to disengage the quad (Figure 5-22).

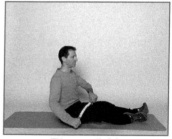

Figure 5-22

- Supporting the back of your pelvis and your lower back by sitting against a wall will help ensure that the quad isn't working to hold the pelvis in place.

- Use the stick along all sides of the quad with as much pressure as you can tolerate, paying specific attention to particularly tender points.

Stretch

Standing Quad Stretch with Support

Stand facing a supportive object, such as a table, wall, chair, or tall foam roller. Place your right hand on the object to stabilize your body.

- Grab your left ankle with your left hand and gently pull your heel up toward your glute (Figure 5-23).

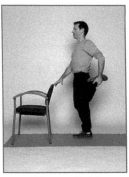

- Your lower back might want to arch to make it easier to bring the foot to the butt. This is your body's compensation for tight quads. DO NOT let this happen.

Figure 5-23

- Bring your foot up until you feel tension in the quad, then hold until it releases. Go a little further if you can. Wait for another release of tension and then move on.

If you cannot reach your ankle to get an effective stretch, you can wrap a towel under your ankle and pull the towel toward your buttocks to feel the stretch in the thigh.

Side-Lying Quad Stretch

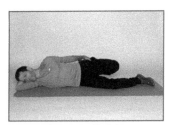

Figure 5-24

- Lie on your side, body perpendicular to the floor, top leg stacked evenly on the bottom leg.

- Bend the lower leg slightly to disengage that quad.

- Relax the top leg and gently pull that ankle towards your glute (Figure 5-24). Do not arch your back to reach the foot. If needed, use a towel, as described in the Standing Quad Stretch.

- Do not allow your hips to rotate. Keep your body straight and hips "stacked" on top of each other.

Strength

Seated Leg Raise

This is similar to the Lying-Straight Leg Raise except that sitting for this action helps move the work from the iliopsoas to the rectus femoris.

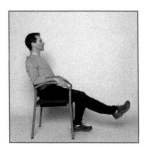

Figure 5-25

- Sit on a chair, with one leg extended straight out. (Figure 5-25)

- If needed, you can lean against the back of the chair for support, as long as you activate your core and keep a neutral spine.

- With control, lift one leg up as far as you comfortably can, then return it to the floor.

- Keep your leg straight throughout the movement, with your toes pointed up.

- The more you slide your butt forward and lean your torso back, the easier the lift.

- Work towards 2 sets of 12 reps.

Back

Fascia Release

When you purchase your foam roller, the instructions will probably show you how to use it on the back muscles. Although this works for some people, I don't suggest doing it without the supervision of an experienced Corrective Exercise Specialist or Personal Trainer.

In order to effectively "roll" the back, you really need to relax into it, and many people find it very difficult to relax into a spinal extension. Also, if you do relax enough, you have to be very careful not to apply too much pressure on your two floating ribs (the bottom two ribs on each side,) as this can cause serious injury. This is why I prefer a ball for this action.

- Stand with your back to a sturdy wall and place a tennis or massage ball between your back and the wall. Make sure there are no switches, plugs or artwork on the wall where you're working (Figure 5-26).

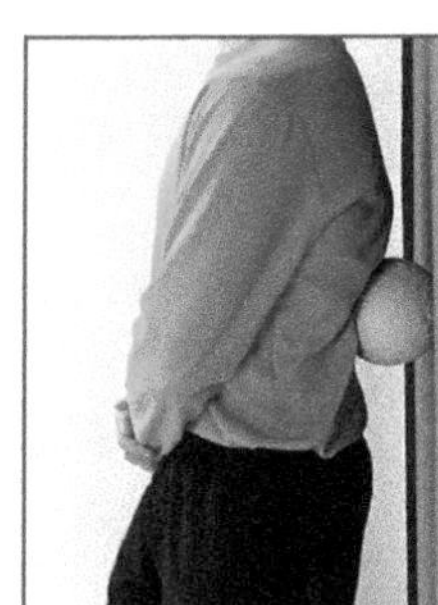

Figure 5-26

- Move your body around while pressing back against the ball. This will require some work from your legs as you bend at the knees to maneuver around the ball.

- Apply whatever pressure you're comfortable with.

- You can safely roll up and down along either side of the spine, from the shoulder area down to the pelvis and glutes.

- Stop and address tender points as per previous instructions.

Although I much prefer using a ball, the back and shoulders are also perfect targets for a Thera Cane. (Figure 5-27) When used as directed, you can get great leverage against the muscles and really isolate the painful points. Although not complicated, effective

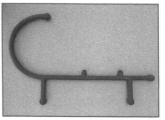

Figure 5-27

directions for the Cane would be tough to accomplish in this manual. If you make the purchase, the images and directions included with the product will make it clear how to take advantage of this great tool.

Stretch

Bend and Reach

Although this action is a bit more complex than many of the others I describe, it's well worth learning.

- Stand facing a supportive surface that is about waist high, such as a chair or table. Place your feet hip or shoulder width apart, put your hands on the support, and pack your shoulders (Figure 5-28).

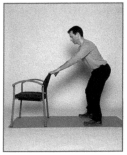 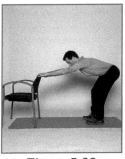 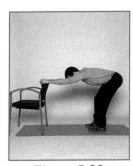

Figure 5-28   Figure 5-29   Figure 5-30

- Stabilize your spine and keep your chest out slightly.

- Bend your knees slightly. Then shift your weight back over your heels and begin slowly bending forward at the hips.

- Keep your arms straight so there is a straight line from the shoulders through the elbows to the wrists (Figure 5-29).

- Lean back into your hips, straighten the legs slightly, if possible (tight hamstrings might make straightening the legs difficult, but don't worry,) and press your torso toward the ground.

- Maintain a straight line from your head through your arms and spine; don't let your head drop towards the floor.

- To increase the stretch, turn your palms up to face the ceiling, while you continue to lean back into your hips.

- Be sure not to "lock" your knees while holding this position.

- Hold until the tension releases. Go deeper if you can, then move on.

Child's Pose

For this action, do the best you can according to your own range of motion.

- Get on your hands and knees on the floor, with your toes pointing behind you and big toes touching if possible.

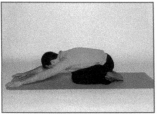

Figure 5-31
Child's Pose

- Spread your knees towards the outside and sit back on your heels.

- As you sit back, try to bring your hips/butt as far back as possible while stretching out your back and arms by reaching along the ground in front of you.

- Lower your chest as far down between your thighs as is comfortable.

- Take a deep breath and then exhale as you lengthen the spine, extending through the upper body, and continuing deeper into the pose, widening your knees as needed.

- Hold this position for 5–10 slow, deep breaths and then move on.

Strength

Superman

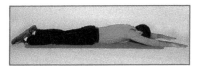

Figure 5-32

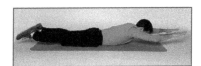

Figure 5-33

- Lie on your stomach with your legs outstretched and your toes pointing towards the wall behind you. Reach your arms out in front of you with your palms facing down or facing each other (Figure 5-32).

- Relax your neck and align your head with your spine.

- Exhale, stabilize your core, and slowly—*with control*—reach both legs away from your torso until they lift a few inches off of the floor. At the same time, raise both arms a few inches off of the floor. Keep your legs and arms straight (Figure 5-33).

- Do not allow your head to lift up or to droop toward the floor; keep it aligned with your spine.

- Hold this position for a count of 2 seconds.

- Hold your breath for the count or breathe through pursed lips.

- Gently relax and—*with control*—lower your legs and arms back to the starting position. Do not allow any extra movement in your low back or hips.

- Work towards two sets of 12 reps.

This exercise is easier when done with alternating leg and arm lifts instead of all four limbs at the same time. For example, lift your left arm and right leg, then lower them, and then do the same for the opposite arm and leg.

Bird Dog

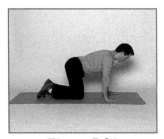

Figure 5-34

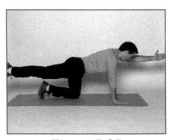

Figure 5-35

- Get on your hands and knees, with your knees under your hips and your wrists directly under your shoulders. Your fingers should be pointing forward. (Figure 5-34)

- Activate your core, stabilize your spine and make

sure there's no excessive sagging or arching in the lower back.

- Start by just trying to lengthen a single leg all the way out behind you until it is parallel to the floor.

- Make sure your glutes are engaged.

- Do not lift the leg above your hips and don't let it go so high as to cause your pelvis to rotate.

- As you feel more confident and balanced, try to slowly raise and straighten the opposite arm (left foot with right arm) until it is parallel or nearly parallel to the floor. Make sure your shoulders remain parallel to the floor (Figure 5-35, page 121).

- Keep your head aligned with your spine throughout the movement.

- Hold the extended position for a count of 2 seconds. Then gently—*with control*—lower yourself back to the starting position. Alternate sides and repeat for a single set of 12 on each side. Add a set as you gain strength and confidence.

- As you alternate sides, keep your core active and try to switch sides with minimal weight shift.

Hamstrings

Fascia Release

- Sit on the floor with one leg straight out in front of you, the other either slightly off to the side (as shown in Figure 5-36) or bent with knee up and foot flat on the floor.

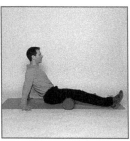

Figure 5-36

- Place the foam roller under the straight leg and, using your arms, roll your body back and forth over the roller.

- The bent leg (with its foot flat on the floor) can be used to help you roll back and forth.

- Lean back as much as you'd like, so long as the core stays active and your back stays lengthened and straight.

- Roll from your glute to just before the back of the knee.

- Do not roll directly behind the knee.

- Do each leg for 1–2 minutes.

You can also get an effective hamstring fascia release with a self-massage stick (Figure 5-37).

- Sit comfortably on the floor and simply roll the stick along your hamstrings with an amount of pressure that's tolerable.

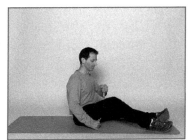

Figure 5-37

- You're able to control the pressure very effectively and move the stick all around the upper leg. It might, however, be a little tougher to address the tender spots than if you used a foam roller.

Stretch

Sitting Hamstring Stretch

You want to make sure your back is straight during this action so you're not gaining movement by flexing the spine. This helps to ensure that you're isolating the hamstrings.

- Sit on the floor with one leg stretched out in front of you and the other slightly bent, so that the bottom of your foot faces the straightened leg. (Figure 5-38, next page) You only need to bend the leg enough to disengage the hamstrings on the bent leg.

- Put your hands on the ground behind or beside you to help support your posture, if needed.

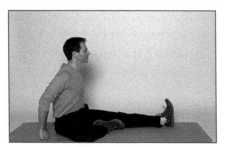

Figure 5-38

- As you exhale, slowly lean forward from your hips.

- It's possible that you'll feel a stretch just by getting into the starting position.

- If this is the case, you don't have to lean forward. Just hold the stretch when you feel it.

- Keep the knee of the stretched leg straight and toes pointed towards the ceiling.

- You don't want to feel a stretch directly behind the knee, as there are no muscles to be worked. If you feel tension behind your knee, reduce the lean a little. This should move the tension back to your hamstring.

Standing Hamstring Stretch with Support

This is a trickier stretch to do correctly than many people think. Remember that while standing or leaning forward the hamstrings go to work to help keep us upright. And if you keep in mind how difficult it is to stretch a muscle that's being used you can see why stretching a hamstring while standing can be a bit tricky. I've included it here, however, because it's a move that so many people are familiar with and, when done right, can be very effective.

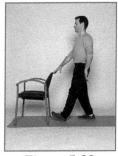

Figure 5-39

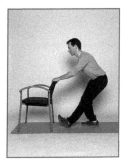

Figure 5-40

- Stand facing a table, a stable chair, or a wall for support. Make sure you're close enough to the support to use it while keeping good posture. (Figure 5-39)

- Place your hands on the support, then step one foot back 12 inches or so and slightly bend your back knee. Keep your back foot flat on the ground while coming up onto the heel of the front foot.

- You'll be stretching the front leg.

- If you feel a stretch at this point, hold until it releases. If not, slowly lean your torso forward, while keeping your spine stabilized. (Figure 5-40) This may require bending your back knee a little more.

- It's very important to take the workload off the front leg by using the support and your back leg to hold your weight.

- Alternate sides when you are ready to do so.

Strength

Bridge

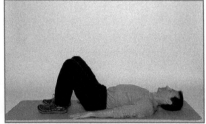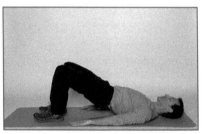

Figure 5-41   Figure 5-42

- Breathing through pursed lips may be helpful for this action.

- Lie on your back with knees bent, feet flat on the floor and arms by your sides, palms down. Make sure your feet are about hip-width apart, with your toes facing straight ahead (Figure 5-41).

- Stabilize your pelvis and lower back, activate your glutes and, while you exhale, lift your hips off the floor by pressing both feet into the ground.

- Your shoulders should stay on the ground for support. Do not rise up onto your head.

- Raise your hips just enough to create a straight line from your knees to your shoulders (Figure 5-42).

- Hold for a count of 2 seconds. Then slowly—*with control*—lower yourself back to your starting position while inhaling.

- Work towards 2 sets of 12 reps.

You can make this exercise a little more difficult by bringing your feet closer together or placing them farther out in front of you. Not completely lowering your back to the floor at the end of each rep can also increase the difficulty.

Glutes

Fascia Release

As you experienced the hamstring fascia and back release, you may have already explored this action, seeing as it's so close to those areas. Either tool will work (roller, ball or cane) depending on your preference. I prefer a ball against a wall.

- Stand with your back a few inches away from a flat, smooth wall and place the ball between your lower back and the wall (Figure 5-43, next page).

- Using your legs, roll the ball against your glute while pushing back against the wall. Apply only as much pressure as you can tolerate.

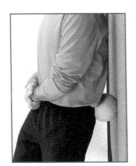

Figure 5-43

- Maneuver the ball all around your glute, including down the sides towards your hips and up to the top of the pelvis.

- Do each side for 1–2 minutes.

If you are using a foam roller on the floor, place it perpendicular to your legs and sit on it. For a deeper release, cross one leg over the opposite knee and focus the roller (or ball) on the glute of the crossed leg.

Stretch

- Lie on your back with your knees bent and feet flat on the ground

- Keep your spine neutral and supported.

- Cross your right leg over your left knee so that your right ankle is resting comfortably on your left thigh (Figure 5-44, next page).

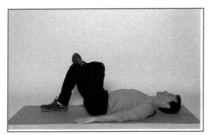 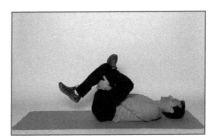

Figure 5-44   Figure 5-45

- If you feel tension in the right glute at this point, that's good. That's the extent of your movement for this stretch.

- If you don't experience tension yet, slowly bring your left knee towards your chest until you feel tension in the right glute. You can gently grab the back of your left (non-stretched) thigh with both hands to help with the movement (Figure 5-45).

- Hold the stretch until the tension releases. Then slowly—*with control*—lower your right foot to the ground and switch legs.

- As always, do not allow your back to arch.

Strength

Standing Hip Extensions

- Stand in good posture in front of a stable surface. Make sure the support is tall enough and close enough that you can reach it easily without bending or leaning forward.

- Maintain a neutral pelvis and lower back while you extend a leg behind you. You may need to bend the leg a bit so it clears the floor as it moves backwards. (Figure 5-46)

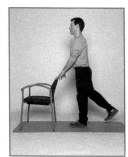

Figure 5-46

- Make sure the non-moving leg stays slightly bent and do not allow your back to arch.

- Return the leg halfway to starting position and repeat for 2 sets of 12 reps for each leg.

   Bird Dog (page 121) and Bridge (page 127) also work well for strengthening the glutes.

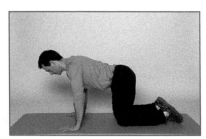
Figure 5-47

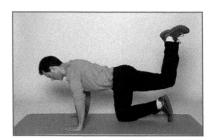
Figure 5-48

Bent Knee Hip Extension

- Get on all fours, with your knees beneath your hips, feet pointing behind you.

- Your hands should be under your shoulders, with your fingers pointing forward (Figure 5-47).

- Make sure your pelvis is neutral and your spine is supported. Do not allow the lower back to sag or arch at all during the movement.

- Lift your left leg, keep the knee bent, and activate the glute while pressing your left foot upward toward the ceiling (Figure 5-48).

- Move only as far as your hip joint allows. Do not move through the pelvis or lower back, or allow your hips to rotate.

- Work towards two sets of 12 reps, each leg.

Final Thoughts

I've given you a lot of information in these pages, but this manual does not substitute, in any way, for a conversation with a qualified health care provider. The goal has been to give you a foundation of knowledge and skills for controlling your low-back pain and now the work is in your hands. It's the practice that keeps it all together— the consistent awareness of body mechanics, along with the discipline of managing muscles and fascia.

My health goals have been simple and straightforward over the past several years: I just want to add more quality to whatever years I have left and hopefully add more healthy years, as well. Underneath that is the desire for the kind of endurance that allows me to keep going and provides the strength to participate in any activity. Learning to manage my low-back pain has had a tremendously positive impact. And now, any project of yard work, furniture moving, or— most importantly—playing with my daughter, gives me the chance to put these techniques to work and to stay strong.

If you make use of these lessons and combine them with a commitment to your own personal health education, awareness of body mechanics, and muscle management, then you can make a significant and immediate difference in your own life. When you feel a twinge or spasm threaten in your lower back, just come back to what you've learned in this manual.

Above all else, keep moving. It's what a body needs to become healthy and stay that way. Check in often to make sure your core is active. Adjust your posture and stand tall and confident, knowing that you can now finally take control of your low-back pain.

Appendix:
Summary of Actions from Lesson Five

All the actions in Lesson Five should be included in an exercise program to help ensure that your muscles are well balanced and functioning at their best. Keep in mind, however, that I've only offered the most basic actions, in order to make this manual accessible to the greatest number of people. For the many beginners who might be seeing some of these actions for the first time, have confidence that this was all designed for use in your home, with no special experience or assistance needed.

For both beginner and experienced exercisers, please remember that there are hundreds of exercise variations out there for keeping your core strong and balanced. Some of them may make sense based on everything you've learned in this manual; some may not, and others you just might not be sure about. As you explore and advance to more difficult exercises, keep this manual in mind. Remember that every action needs to start with an active core and continue with proper mechanics.

If you come across a resource that suggests a deviation from that one simple rule, then strongly question it. Find out the reasons behind the instructions you are being given. If someone from a gym does not include core activation and stability as part of your instruction for a particular action, walk away and find someone else.

These final few pages contain a general summary of the important points of Lesson Five. First, I highlight some important guidelines for organizing your exercises. Second, I describe all of the actions with only images and a few key points. This might be helpful if all you need are reminders of what works for which muscles. Make full use of all of the information and never forget to keep your core active and spine supported for *all* the movements.

For the best results, do fascia release first, stretch next, then strengthen.

- You can choose to do *all* the self-massage actions first, then *all* the stretches, etc. But you can also massage, stretch, and then strengthen a specific location, after which you move on to another location and continue in that way. It's your choice.

- Unless otherwise noted, fascia release exercises can be just 1-2 minutes in duration, depending on your tolerance and stamina, and can be done each day.

- All of the strength exercises described in this manual can be done every day, but should be done no less than 3 times per week.

- Rest for at least 1 or 2 minutes between sets of any given strength exercise, unless otherwise noted.

- All of the actions in this lesson should be included in an exercise program, but in any instance where I've offered more than one massage, stretch or strength action for a particular muscle, you only need to choose one (plank and crunch are the exceptions—do both).

- Talk to your doctor to discuss any exercise routine.

Abdominal

Fascia Release

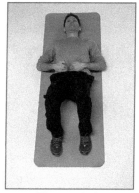

The best use of this action is when your pain level is high. It can work very well if you've just had a full-blown "back attack" or one is threatening.

Figure A-1
Fascia Release

Stretch

This is the Standing Stretch and Cobra for the rectus abdominis. It has a slight twist during the standing stretch that will work the obliques. Remember Cobra may not work for everyone so, if you feel no stretch during this move or it's too strenuous, just move on.

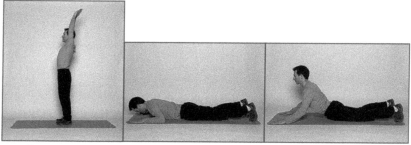

Figure A-2
Standing Strech

Figure A-4
Cobra

Strength

Crunches are for the rectus and obliques (add a slight twist while raising up to work the obliques) and planks focus the work more specifically on the TVA.

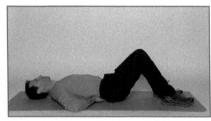 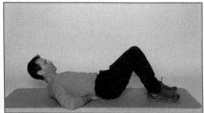

Figure A-3, Crunch

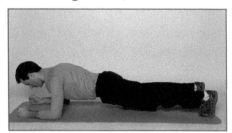

Figure A-4, Plank

Hip Flexor—Iliacus and psoas (iliopsoas)

Fascia Release

This is very similar to the abdominal fascia release and can easily be done at the same time. Figures A-6 and A-7 shows the iliacus release.

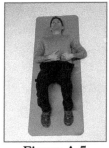 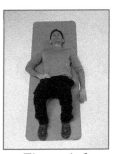 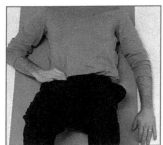

Figure A-5	Figure A-6	Figure A-7
Psoas Release	Iliacus Release	Iliacus Release, Closeup

Stretch

This stretch effects both the iliopsoas and rectus femoris. A lunge with an overhead reach focuses the stretch more on the psoas. If you add a very slight twist onto the forward leg, you'll get more activity in the iliacus.

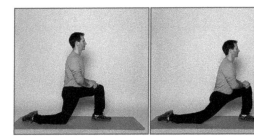 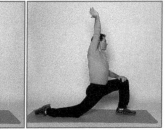

Figure A-8, Lunge Stretch

Strength

Make sure your spine is well supported for this action. If you feel your lower back straining, stop the exercise. This means your core is not able to give you enough support for the move. Build a little more core strength and try it again in a week or so.

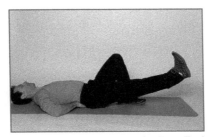

Figure A-9, Lying-Straight Leg Raise

Hip Flexor—Rectus Femoris

Fascia Release

Do not roll directly over the kneecap.

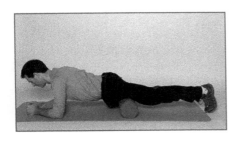
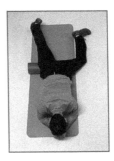

Figure A-10
Fascia
Release,
Foam Roller

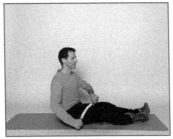

Figure A-11: Fascia Release, Massage Stick

Stretch

Make sure your weight is well supported and balanced during the standing quad stretch, and that you're not arching your lower back during either stretch.

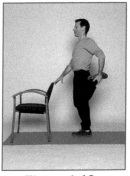

Figure A-12
Standing Quad Stretch
with Support

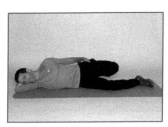

Figure A-13
Side-Lying Quad Stretch

Strength

This is similar to the lying straight leg raise except that sitting for this action helps move the work from the iliopsoas to the rectus femoris. The further you lean back, the easier the move will be.

Figure A-14
Seated Leg Raise

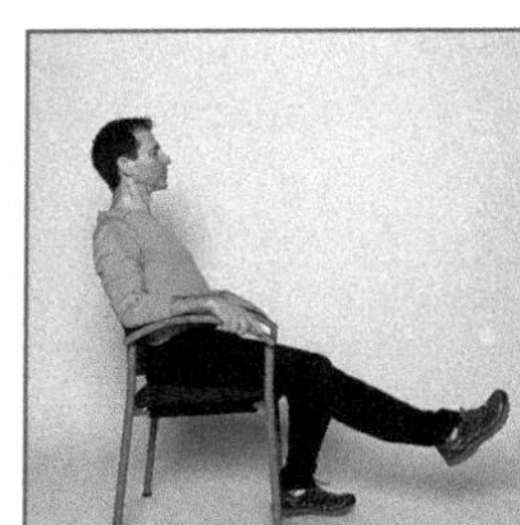

Back

Fascia Release

This can be done up and down the entire back, through the shoulders and into the glutes but please do not roll directly over your spine.

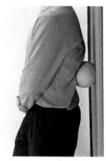

Figure A-15
Fascia Release

Stretch

You can increase the effect of the Bend and Reach by pushing your glutes further back. For the Child's Pose, go only as far forward as your range of motion allows.

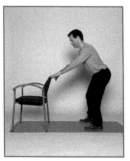 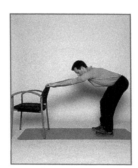 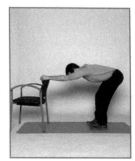

Figure A-16, Bend and Reach

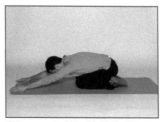

Figure A-17, Child's Pose

Strength

The Superman can be strenuous for beginners and it might be best to start with the alternating arm/leg version, as described on page 121. The Bird Dog action is a great alternative, but remember to keep your hips level and be careful to keep your core active during transition from one side to the other.

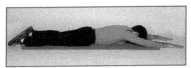 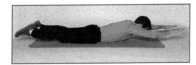

Figure A-18, Superman

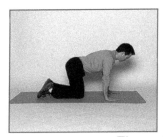 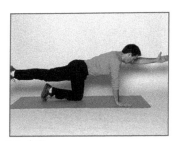

Figure A-19, Bird Dog

Hamstrings

Fascia Release

It's very common to roll or use a stick on the hamstrings while doing the quads.

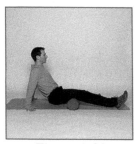 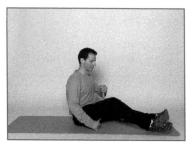

Figure A-20, Hamstring Fascia Release with
Roller and Massage Stick

Stretch

The Sitting Hamstring Stretch can be done with both legs at the same time, but I think the single leg action improves the effectiveness for each leg. Make sure you are well supported and balanced for the Standing Hamstring Stretch.

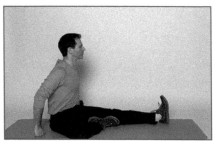

Figure A-21
Sitting Hanstring Stretch

Figure A-22
Standing Hamstring
Stretch

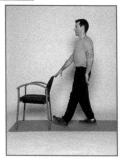 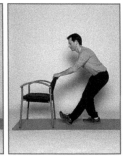

Strength

The Bridge will work the glutes and TVA, as well as the hamstrings. To increase the difficulty, try moving your feet further out in front of you.

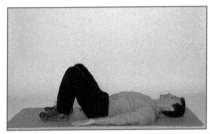 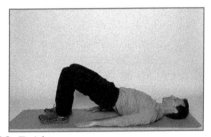

Figure A-23, Bridge

Glutes

Fascia Release

You can do this while also doing the low-back.

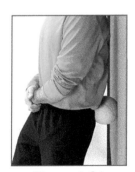

Figure A-24
Glutes Fascia Release

Stretch

Make sure your back doesn't arch during this stretch.

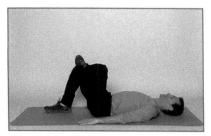 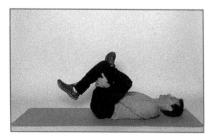

Figure A-25, Glutes Stretch

Strength

It is important to keep your lower back and pelvis neutral during the Standing Hip Extension. This means that the motion extends only as far backward as you can go before the back needs to arch to allow further movement. Stay focused on keeping the spine neutral and hips level during the Bent Knee Extension.

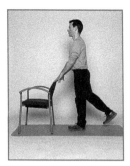

Figure A-26, Standing Leg Extenstion

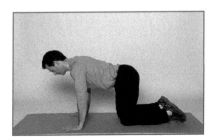 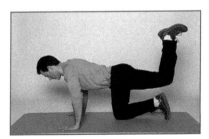

Figure A-27, Bent Knee Extension

Works Cited

Adams, M. A., S. May, B. J. Freeman, H. P. Morrison, and P. Dolan, (2000). Effects of backward bending on lumbar intervertebral discs. Relevance to physical therapy treatments for low back pain. *Spine, 25* (4), 431-437.

Allison, G., S. Morris, and B. Lay. (2008). *Journal of Orthopaedic & Sports Physical Therapy, 38* (5), 228-237.

American Chiropractic Association. *Back Pain Facts and Statistics.* Retrieved May 2, 2015, from http://www. acatoday.org/Patients/Health-Wellness-Information/ Back-Pain-Facts-and-Statistics

American Council on Exercise (2010). *ACE's Essentials of Exercise Science for Fitness Professionals.* (C. X. Brayant and D. J. Green, eds.) San Diego, CA: American Council on Exercise.

Briñol, Pablo, Richard E. Petty, and Benjamin Wagner (2009). Body posture effects on self-evaluation: A self-validation approach. *European Journal of Social Psychology,* 39 (6), 1053-1064.

Cailliet, Rene and Leonard Gross. (1987). *Rejuvenation Strategy.* New York, NY: Doubleday.

Chiro Economics. (2010, February). *Top 5 consequences to bad posture.* Retrieved from Chiroeco.com

Deardorff, William W. PhD, ABPP (2003, March 11). *The Gate Control Theory of Modern Pain.* Retrieved from spine-health.com:http://www.spine-health.com/conditions/chronic-pain/gate-control-theory-chronic-pain-action

Dodge, Phil DC. (2015, July 1). Facet joint anatomy and function. [Personal interview].

Dunstan, David W., Alicia A. Thorp, and Genevieve N. Healy. "Prolonged Sitting." *Current Opinion in Cardiology* 26.5 (2011): 412-19. Web.

Hoy, D., P. Brooks, F. Blyth and R. Buchbinder. (2010, December). The epidemiology of low back pain. *Best Practice & Research Clinical Rheumatology*, 769-781.

Hoy, D., L. March, P. Brooks, A, Woolf, C. Bain, G. Williams, et al. (2014, March). The Global Burden of Low Back Pain: Estimates from the Global Burden of Disease 2010 Study. *Annals of the Rheumatic Diseases*, 968-974.

Huether, Sue E. and Kathryn L. McCance, (2004). *Understanding Pathophysiology* (3rd edition). St. Louis, MO: Mosby.

IASP Taxonomy. International Association for the Study of Pain, 22 May 2012. Web. 24 May 2015. http://www.iasp-pain.org/Taxonomy#Pain

Kapandji, I. A. (2008). *The Physiology of the Joints* (6th ed.). Edinburgh: Churchill Livingstone/Elsevier.

Koyama, Tetsuo, John G. McHaffie, Paul J. Laurienti, and Robert C. Coghill (2005). The subjective experience of pain: Where expectations become reality. (E. E. Smith, Ed.) Proceedings of the National Academy of Sciences of the United States of America, 102 (36), 12950–12955.

Matthews, C., S. George, S. Moore, H. Bowles, A. Blair, Y. Park, A. Schatzkin. (2012). Amount of time spent in sedentary behaviors and cause-specific mortality in US adults. *American Journal of Clinical Nutrition,* 437-445.

McGill, Stuart. (2007). *Low Back Disorders: Evidence-based Prevention and Rehabilitation.* (Second Edition.) Champaign, IL: Human Kinetics.

McGill, Stuart. *Spine flexion exercise: Myths, Truths and Issues affecting health and performance.* Retrieved from Backfitpro.com: http://www.backfitpro.com/documents/Spine-flexion-myths-truths-and-issues.pdf

Melzack, R., and P. D. Wall (1965). Pain Mechanisms: A New Theory. *Science, 150* (3699), 971-979.

Merriam-Webster. *Spasm defined.* Retrieved from Merriam-Webster.com: http://www.merriam-webster.com/dictionary/spasm

Moffat, Marilyn and Steve Vickery (1999). *American Physical Therapy Association Book of Body Maintenance and Repair.* New York, NY: Henry Holt.

Nachemson, A. L. (1981). Disc pressure measurements. *Spine, 6* (1), 93-97.

National Institute of Neurological Disorders and Stroke. (2014, December). *Low Back Pain Fact Sheet.* Retrieved December 2014, from National Institute of Neurological Disorders and Stroke: http://www.ninds.nih.gov/disorders/backpain/ detail_backpain.htm#3102_4

Nelson, Arnold G. and Jouko Kokkonen. (2007). *Stretching anatomy.* Champaign, IL: Human Kinetics.

Ponte, David Joseph, MA, PT, Gail J. Jensen, MA, PT and Barbara E. Kent, MA, PT (1984, Sep/Oct). A preliminary report on the use of the McKenzie protocol versus Williams protocol in the treatment of low back pain. *Journal of Orthopaedic & Sports Physical Therapy,* 130-139.

Price, Justin (2009). *Understanding Muscles and Movement.* Space Café Media.

Radcliff, Kristen E. MD, Christopher K. Kepler, MD, Andre Jakoi, MD, Gursukhman S. Sidhu, MBBS, Jeffery Rihn, MD, Alexander R. Vaccaro, MD, PhD, Todd J. Albert,

MD, Alan S. Hilibrand, MD (2013). Adjacent segment disease in the lumbar spine following different treatment interventions. *The Spine Journal, 13* (10), 1339–1349.

Woolf, Anthony D. and Bruce Pfleger (2003). Burden of major musculoskeletal conditions. *Bulletin of the World Health Organization, 81*, p. 652.

Bibliography

A Step-by-Step Guide to Using the NIOSH Lifting Equation for Single Tasks—Ergonomics Plus. (2012, December 5). Retrieved August 10, 2014.

Acute vs. Chronic Pain. (2014, July 7). Retrieved September 20, 2015.

Agus, David B. MD (2012). *The End of Illness*. New York: Free Press.

Back Pain, Neck Pain, Lower Back Pain, and Spinal Disorders by Spine Experts | SpineUniverse. Retrieved February 18, 2015.

Bordoni, Bruno,and Emiliano Zanier (2013). Skin, Fascias, and Scars: Symptoms and Systemic Connections. *Journal of Multidisciplinary Healthcare, 7,* 11-24. doi:10.2147/JMDH. S52870

Boyle, Kyndall L., PT, PhD, OCS, PRC, Josh Olinick, DPT, MS, and Cynthia Lewis PT, PhD (2010). The Value of Blowing up a Balloon. *North American Journal of Sports Physical Therapy, 5*(3), 179-188.

Bryant, Cedric X., PhD and Sabrena Merrill, MS (Ed.). (2013). *ACE health coach manual: The ultimate guide to wellness, fitness, and lifestyle change* (First ed.). San Diego, CA: American Council on Exercise.

Chaffin, Don B., Andersson, Gunnar B. J., and Martin, Bernard J. (1999). *Occupational Biomechanics* (3rd ed.). New York: Wiley.

Cotton, Richard T. (Ed.). (1996). *Personal Trainer Manual:The Resource for Fitness Professionals* (2nd ed.). San Diego, Calif.: American Council on Exercise.

Delavier, Frederic, Jean-Pierre Clemenceau, and Michael Gundill (2011). *Delavier's Stretching Anatomy.* Champaign, IL: Human Kinetics.

Delavier, Frederic (2001). *Strength Training Anatomy* (Vol. 1 & 2). Champaign, IL: Human Kinetics.

Dreyer, Danny and Katherine Dreyer (2004). *ChiRunning: A Revolutionary Approach to Effortless, Injury-Free Running.* New York: Simon & Schuster.

Ferriss, Timothy (2010). *The 4Hour Body: An Uncommon Guide to Rapid Fat Loss, Incredible Sex, and Becoming Superhuman.* New York: Crown Archetype.

Ingraham, Paul and Tim Taylor, MD, (2015, February 1). Trigger Points and Myofascial Pain. A guide to the unfinished science of muscle pain, with reviews of every theory and self-treatment and therapy option. Retrieved March 8, 2015.

Lieberman, Daniel (2013). *The Story of the Human Body: Evolution, Health, and Disease.* New York: Vintage Books.

Marshall, P., and Murphy, D. (2003). The validity and reliability of surface EMG to assess the neuromuscular response of the abdominal muscles to rapid limb movement. *Journal of Electromyography and Kinesiology, 13*(5), 477-489. doi:10.1016/S1050- 6411(03)00027-0

McCall, Pete. "Cutting Edge: Training the Fascial Network (Parts 1and 2)." Acefitness.org. The American Council on Exercise. Web.

McGrath, Chris. "Fit Life / Why You Should Be Foam Rolling." ACE Fitness. The American Council on Exercise, Web.

Moayedi, Massieh and Karen D. Davis (Jan 2013). Theories of pain: from specificity to gate control. *Journal of Neurophysiology, 109* (1), 5-12.

Myers, Thomas (2011). Fascial Fitness: Training in the Neuromyofascial Web. *Idea Fitness Journal, 8*(4).

Price, Derrick MS. (2014). Somatic Health: What do you need to know about training the myofascial lines? *IDEA Mind-Body Wellness Review, 1*(1).

Punnett, L., Prüss-Ütün, A., Nelson, D.I., Fingerhut, M.A., Leigh, J., Tak, S., and Phillips, S. (2005). Estimating the global burden of low back pain attributable to combined occupational exposures. *Am. J. Ind. Med. American Journal of Industrial Medicine,* 459-469. Retrieved July 24, 2014, from http://www.who.int/ quantifying_ehimpacts/global/5lowbackpain.pdf

Ratey, John J. and Eric Hagerman (2008). *Spark: The Revolutionary New Science of Exercise and the Brain.* New York: Little, Brown.

Stark, Stephen D., MD. (1999). *The Stark Reality of Stretching: An Informed Approach for All Activities and Every Sport* (Rev. & expanded 4th ed.). Richmond, B.C.: Stark Reality.

NOTES

CPSIA information can be obtained
at www.ICGtesting.com
Printed in the USA
LVHW012029080419
613326LV00027B/1144/P